# Perfect Posture

**Why Posture is Not Perfect**

**What Perfect Posture Is**

**What Perfect Posture Can Do**

**How to Get Perfect Posture**

**How to Keep Perfect Posture**

# David Paul, R.N.

**Drawings
By Mark Monlux**

**△ Trafford**
PUBLISHING®  www.trafford.com

**North America & international**
toll-free: 844-688-6899 (USA & Canada)
fax: 812 355 4082

There was a young man from the city
Who stood how he should, oh so pretty
But as he grew old his body did fold
Decrepit and bent, what a pity.

This man should have known
His culture had thrown
His backbone out with fashion's ditty.

# Table of

# Contents

# Preface

Thirty years ago, without forethought or knowledge of modern medicine, circumstance set me on a course to become a Registered Nurse. Within five years of graduation from school I found myself with a severe, immobilizing back injury. Thus began a 25-year study of the available literature and observation of generations of clients as well as personal experience and experiment. What had started as an attempt to fix my back evolved into a comprehensive study of the way the human body works as a whole.

After 25 years, I've found nothing to contradict or disprove the principles presented in this postural owner's manual for the human body. So I don't think I'm rushing into print. I believe this is the most understandable explanation of the dynamics of posture you will find.

Therefore, I introduce these principles and methodologies of body mechanics with a high degree of confidence in their accuracy, safety and predictability of outcome. I think you will find the logic and soundness of the views persuasive and understandable, regardless of your education or background.

— David Paul, RN

# Introduction

With Perfect Posture body mechanics you are standing in a manner that properly proportions and evenly tones your body – front to back, side to side, from top to bottom. It also enables your body to maintain its optimum functional potential. Posture is not *just* about looking good anymore. Someone once said, "You are what you eat." It is now time to say, "You are how you stand."

What is Perfect Posture? Perfect Posture is the process of maintaining the body in a position of equilibrium of balance. What is meant by the phrase "equilibrium of balance"? Equilibrium is the harmony that results from the balance of contraries. It is the dead center where the opposition of opposing forces – being equal in strength – succeeds in a balanced, resting motion. It is the central point - the point within the circle of physical symmetry. It is the living synthesis of counterbalanced power. I shall refer to this subject again in explaining the Perfect Posture. This doctrine of equilibrium, balance, centering and symmetry is fundamental in the concept of Perfect Posture. I will use these terms interchangeably in reference to Perfect Posture. They mean almost the same thing, and you can't have one without the other.

Perfect Posture or form might be also described as the mid-point between activity and rest. You're using a necessary, balanced amount of each. Take activity away and the body becomes distorted. Take rest away and the body becomes exhausted. Either way the body is compromised or useless. Thus proper posture could be described as active resting or restive action. It's that position where the body is balanced between activity and rest. It's the upright position of alignment where a normal state of continuous slight tension in muscle tissue, called tonus, is coursing evenly through all the muscles of the body. With practice, this position of alignment can be maintained without conscious effort, even while standing and feeling relaxed. It can be maintained while using no more effort than you do with your current way of standing.

It would be incomplete to show what Perfect Posture is without an explanation of why it's Perfect Posture. By the same token, you should know what is not perfect posture and why it's not. In this way, you will understand the complete dynamics of posture and the process of making it perfect. It's always best to understand what you're doing and why. If you don't, you'll be following along with blind faith, reasoning that it's too complicated and someone must be smarter than you. Or you'll think someone has inside knowledge or education that you don't. This book will explain what is Perfect Posture, what is not Perfect Posture – and why. It will be explained in a way that should be understandable to just about anyone. You can then obtain the benefits of getting it and keeping it, confident you understand exactly what you're doing and why. In this book, you'll learn the commandments of how to stand, walk and sit, so your body maintains its form and function as you age. If you're already old, it will show you how to redefine your body to the shape it was in when you were younger. You'll probably be even better, since poor postural habits start at an early age.

This book will be your blueprint to build a lean, sexy, healthy body. You'll learn to feel when you're standing correctly, not hold yourself in a position you think or have been told you ought to. This system of body mechanics, postural biomechanics or structural hygiene, so to speak, will allow you to contour and tone your body without monotonous or strenuous exercises. The argument could even be made that we are allergic to exercise as it makes most, if not all, to be truthful, turn red, sweat and become short of breath. Personally, even though exercise doesn't contain four letters,

I consider it a dirty word.

Some progressions and visualization drills will be shown, but they are by no means mandatory to accomplish Perfect Posture. They can be used to accelerate the process of adjustment and maintain it. The speed of adjustment will be relative to three variables.

**1) Duration and intensity of concentration on the system;**

**2) The amount of adjustment an individual needs;**

**3) The intelligence of an individual because that sort of individual can orient themselves more quickly to a new situation.**

If you're in the military and want to achieve peak human performance, maximize recovery from activity or equipment load and minimize age-related decline in physical performance, practice Perfect Posture.

If you're in an occupation where looks are essential, practice Perfect Posture. It's essential.

If you want to gain one to three inches in height, practice Perfect Posture.

If you're of Asian descent and want to lose the characteristic flat bottom, slumped shoulders, plus gain an inch to three in height, practice Perfect Posture.

If your body seems to have all the right parts, but no tone and exercise in the common sense is unappealing, practice Perfect Posture. You'll get toned.

If you're a woman who is pregnant or may become so and would like to do the least amount of damage to your body as possible, practice Perfect Posture.

If you are obese and are losing some or all of that weight, don't go from obese, soft and disproportionate to slender, soft and disproportionate. Incorporate Perfect Posture into your program. Burn some calories and get your body aligned at the same time. Be slender, properly proportioned and evenly toned, front to back, side to side, from top to bottom – without exercise.

If you are a nurse (can't forget my fellow nurses) and you have an aching, injured back keeping you from performing at your ultimate level, Perfect Posture positioning is the pathway to back repair and healthy spinal hygiene. Fix your back and help your co-workers and patients fix theirs.

How and why all this can and will occur, if you follow instructions, is explained in a non-technical, understandable manner.

Perfect Posture offers the most return for effort on the fitness index of any belt tightening or fat cutting method you will find. Naturally. It's therefore, your best investment in the economy of movement. Naturally. Through concentration and establishment of centered postural habits, you will have a natural calorie-burning tonus continuously running through all the muscles of the body. Naturally. All of the joints in your body will function at the pitch and angle they were created for. This means vastly reduced chances of painful spinal and joint degeneration or inflammation. Naturally. Perfect Posture is and does all of these things, besides giving you an attractive appearance. Therefore, it now seems time to say, "Let your posture be your exercise and your exercise be your posture."

You will find no adrenalin-amped fitness cheerleaders to inspire you to another peak, only to fall into another trough when you tire of the drudgery. No latest piece of equipment, with a number of easy payments, to put in the garage with the others you're already bored with. Perfect Posture is a way of life. Perfect Posture takes the place of a whole gym full of machines. The pieces of equipment are infinitely convenient. They're with you all the time. You can use them anywhere. Better abs, hips, thighs, buns. Better everything. All in two machines: your mind and your body.

What are you waiting for?

Start practicing Perfect Posture.

# Chapter One
# Why Posture Is Not Perfect

## Part One:
## Outside Influences

To understand what Perfect Posture is and how to get it, you should understand why posture is *not* perfect and how it becomes so. This chapter will demonstrate the first half of why posture is not perfect. It will show how "cultural" or "outside" influences encourage behaviors and related positions. These behaviors and positions then become habits. When held continuously, repetitively, or both, these positions alter the body's form. Imperfect posture might be defined as "an alteration in the body's natural form due to birth defect, illness, injury or behavior". Behaviors can include an association with an object or artifact. To keep the scope of the book within reasonable limits, behavior, at times involving an object or artifact, will be the only cause, or causes, covered. This is because behaviors, at times associated with artifacts, are by far the most common causes of body alterations – in other words: poor posture.

In this chapter I'll identify some behaviors, past and present, which were or are responsible for altering the body's form and function. To do this I'll show examples of "cultural" behaviors with associated positions that become habits. These habits cause changes in the body resulting in the loss of natural proportion, evenly toned form, properly functioning joints or a combination of all three. This loss *then* limits the body's ability to painlessly perform at peak potential and appearance.

The cause and effect relationship of these habits is seldom recognized as substantial. These examples will open your eyes to the significance of their effects. A range of cultures will be considered and compared to Western civilization. The object of the comparisons is an increased awareness that cultural habits can, and do, alter the body's form and function. Not just in "other people's" culture but our own as well.

I'll additionally present some examples of cultural artifacts or objects to show how their habitual use can alter the body. You'll be able to see that habitual use of artifacts is also a reason for an unnaturally altered physical appearance and performance.

Cultural habits become entrenched at an early age, so it feels natural to stand in an anatomically incorrect manner as you age. It causes no immediate discomfort or notice. So it's no surprise that the idea of habits causing alterations in the body's form and function is not as plain as the nose in front of your face. You probably seldom picture your nose and what it's doing because you're immersed in your body. You probably seldom picture your cultural habits and what they're doing because you're immersed in everyday activities. I'll hold up some pictures of other cultures next to Western culture. In this way, you can see that all cultures have comparable characteristics that alter the body's natural form. The differences are just a matter of:

1)  **The degree of departure from the natural body position;**
2)  **The rationale for a particular position;**
3)  **The body part or parts affected.**

The list of alterations resulting from these habits is long. It includes bunions, spongy calves, bad knees, cellulite, saddlebags, flabby buttocks, bad back, pinched nerves, protruding abdomen, slouching shoulders and stiff necks to name a few. The list goes on from aches to pains to strains. All or most are due to habitual positioning, at times associated with artifacts. These problems advance slowly and are considered unavoidable, or part of the aging process to a casual or everyday observer.

## Form Altering Habits

### *Holding* the body

An example of a habit causing an alteration might be seen in the Hindu holy men of India. One might lock or *hold* an arm upright for years as a means of attaining enlightenment or realization of their fundamental unity with God. Eventually, the arm is altered. [Image 1.01] It withers away and becomes useless. People there might admire how straight and tall the man's arm is. In Hindu culture this habit and its effect would be looked upon as a sign of virtue. To someone not immersed in East Indian culture, the withered arm would seem an oddity. It would be looked at as something that could be corrected with time and concentration. In other words, within certain limits, if it were allowed to relax, the arm would eventually drop to his side and regain its natural form and function. With some stretching and gentle exercise, it might resume its natural form and function more quickly. Recovery would be relative to the amount of time and concentration devoted and how long and intensely his arm had been in the upheld position. But, it would cause pain to lower it too rapidly, possibly causing irreparable damage. It would have to be returned to a natural position and function slowly. Ligaments can pull or tear if manipulated too forcefully. (Remember this when engaging in the progressions outlined later in this book. Don't go too fast. You can irreparably damage yourself. You could get discouraged and return to your previous, unnatural way of standing, walking and sitting. A more in-depth explanation of the reasons for adjusting slowly and gently will be addressed in the progression chapter.)

An example of a comparable form altering habit in Western culture exists. Consider the widespread habit of locking or *holding* the knees to the rear. Couple this with locking or *holding* our upper bodies in a "chin up, chest out, stomach in, shoulders back" position. [Image 1.02] This is

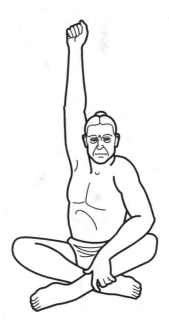

**Image 1.01**
**A Hindu holy man holding his arm over his head.**

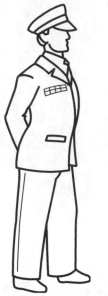

**Image 1.02**
A man locking his knees back, holding the chin up, chest out, stomach in, shoulders back, "Up Straight " position.

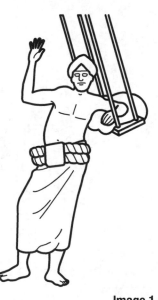

**Image 1.03**
A Hindu holy man on one foot.

done to show respect or to look respectable. People might remark how straight, tall and striking the position appears. In an attempt to **always** look respectable, this becomes the way most people **always** stand. The eventual slouch of the shoulders, hunchback, over-arched low back and numerous other significant physical alterations this habit causes are comparable to the significant alteration of the holy man's arm.

For whatever reason, locking the knees back and *holding* the "chin up, chest out, stomach in, shoulders back" position is not widely recognized as a body altering habit. But it is, as will be shown. (As with the Hindu man's arm, it will require the same precautions to properly reposition the back and other body parts this habit alters.)

In this example:

1) **The degree of departure from the body's natural position is about equal;**
2) **The rationale for holding the bodies in these positions is different;**
3) **The body part or parts affected is different but the consequences are profound in both cases. The Hindu man's arm becomes withered and useless. The Western man's spine becomes crooked and dysfunctional.**

**Resting on one foot**

A Hindu individual may lock the knee back and stand on one foot for years at a time. [Image 1.03] The reason for the behavior would again be a desire for enlightenment. Eventually, this will cause not only an over-arched front-to-back curvature to the waist level spine, but also a side-to-side curvature. In Hindu culture, this side-to-side spinal alteration would be looked upon as a sign of an honorable individual. In Western culture, it would be considered a disease process and defined as scoliosis.

There is a comparable example to be seen in western civilization. It's the habit of standing, possibly in an exaggerated manner, with the body's weight being supported on one leg with the knee locked back. [Image 1.04] The motivating factor in this instance is a desire to look attractive or confident. This also causes an over-arched waist level spine and side-to-side curvature. Though usually not as severe because most do not stand this way continuously, it does have an effect and can become significant. This is especially so if someone develops the habit of standing on one side only. (Fifteen minutes spent bearing weight on one locked-up leg per day = ninety-one hours or almost four days per year. That's more than a month per decade. That's close to a year in a 70-year-old lifetime and more than enough time to cause a significant alteration to a body.) The eventual spinal alterations are commonly thought of as part of "getting old." It simply does not occur to most that the way you stand and the body's noteworthy reactions to it are related to each other.

In this example:

1)  **The degree of departure from the natural or balanced body position is about the same in both cultures;**
2)  **The rationale for holding the bodies in these positions is different;**
3)  **The body part, or parts, affected is identical. Basically, it has the same effect: an overarched waist level back and sideways curvature of the spine.**

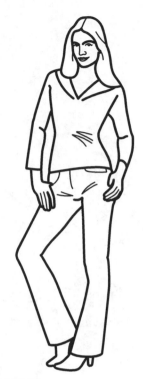

**Image 1.04**
**Woman posturing on one foot to look attractive or confident.**

## Habitual Use of Artifacts

### Foot binding and pointy shoes

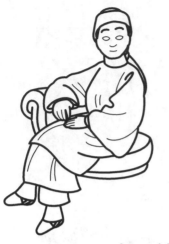

**Image 1.05**
**Chinese woman with bound feet.**

To compare the effects of an artifact, consider the one-time tradition of foot binding in China. [Image 1.05] At an early age, women's feet were bound with cloth to stop them from growing more than four inches or so. Normal, big feet were considered alien to feudal virtues. If you were to ask these women why they subjected themselves to these artifacts and the resultant departure from the natural form they would probably say, "What departure?" They wouldn't recognize the deformity, associated poor balance and lowered bone density as anything but the normal results of the aging process. The awkward gait wouldn't seem unusual or funny because everyone walked that way. Or they might answer, "Yes, I understand, but it's the price you pay to look good."

It's not too big a mental leap to compare these practices and artifacts to the high heeled, pointy toe shoes fashionable in our society. If you asked a westerner why they wear those kinds of shoes you would get pretty much the same response as from the Chinese. The cause and effect relationship of the artifacts also would be unrecognized or tolerated for the sake of acceptance by associates. Foot binding in China is now looked upon as a form of subjugation and mutilation. In the future will we look at high-heeled pointy shoes in the same way? [Image 1.06]

In this example:

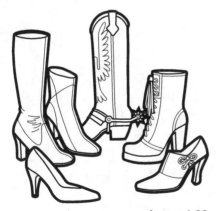

**Image 1.06**
**High heels are an example of an artifact enhancing the effects of the locked back knees, "Up Straight" position.**

1) **The degree of departure from the natural body position is more severe with foot binding;**
2) **The rationale for having held, or holding, the bodies in these positions is similar;**
3) **The body part or parts affected is identical. The gait is altered in both instances.**

## Headboards and straight-backed chairs

The Flathead Indians of America applied a board to the forehead at an early age. [Images 1.07] It created a characteristic by which they became identified as a people. This practice was discouraged by Western Europeans and disappeared. What came with the Europeans was the straight-backed, upright chair. A comparison can be made. The use of the Indian headboard caused an unnaturally straightened forehead. It's comparable to the use of straight-backed chairs which were, and are, meant to cause a (*unnaturally*) straightened back. [Image 1.08] The words "meant to" are used because it didn't – and doesn't – work. Consistently sitting too straight is one of the main reasons for the slouching shoulders, swayback lower spine and low-back problems we see so much of today. It has the opposite of its intended effect. These effects are again commonly referred to as the "aging process." The straight-backed chair is not widely recognized as a form-altering device in Western culture – but it is, as will be shown.

There is a difference between the effects of the practices on foreheads and backs. The forehead cannot be reshaped once the forehead is mature. The back is jointed, more flexible and can resume a natural curvature with proper conditioning at almost any age. But, you can see the relation of an artifact to body modification. The forehead was not created to be straightened by a headboard any more than the backbone by a straight-backed chair. In this example:

1) **The degree of departure from the natural body position seems about equal. It's profound in both. It's difficult to precisely compare foreheads with backs;**
2) **The rationales for the positioning are questionable but possibly the same (to look attractive, or respectable?);**
3) **The body part affected is different.**

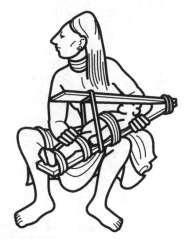

**Image 1.07**
**Flathead Indian and child.**

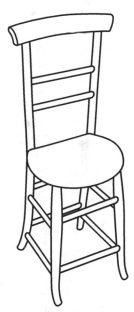

**Image 1.08**
**Edwardian straightback chair.**

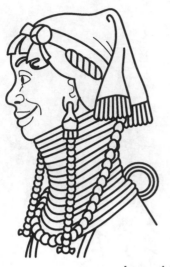

**Image 1.09**
**Burmese woman with neck rings.**

## Balanced Healing

I'll compare one example of habits and artifacts compromising the body's ability to maintain equilibrium and, therefore, health. The purpose of this comparison is different from the others. The object of this comparison is to show that symmetry and balance within a body and knowing how to find it on an internal level is important. It's important so a body can safely achieve maximum recovery in minimal time, perform at optimum level and not wear out prematurely. Symmetry, balance and knowing how to find it will be shown in Chapter 2.

Balanced muscle strength is the ability of a pair of muscles on either side of a fulcrum or pivot in the body to be equally strong on both sides. Examples would be the front-to-back, side-to-side muscles of the neck or back. If muscles become stronger on one side of the body and weaker on the other it can cause an alteration in the shape of the spine. This then can cause pinched nerves, numbness, tingling, blurred vision, pain and possibly debility. Without knowing how to find the Perfect Posture, or balanced position, recovery may unknowingly be slowed, complicated or even prevented.

Consider the women of the Padaung tribe in Asia who wear rings on their neck to extend its length. [Image 1.09] They keep adding rings. It adds to beauty and respect. They might consider their debilitating neck, back and shoulder problems part of the price you pay for beauty. If the rings were taken away for some reason and the neck had not been stretched too long, it could eventually resume its natural contour. They would need to take care and hold the head correctly balanced on the shoulders to establish balanced muscle strength. Balanced muscle strength would maximize recovery. It would ensure the head wouldn't habitually lean too far this way or that, and injure the nerve roots in its altered state.

The equipment and activity loads from some of the increasingly sophisticated headgear worn by modern ground troops, tank crews, jet and helicopter pilots is a comparable artifact. [Image 1.10] These artifacts and activities can compromise the neck's ability to maintain proper position and balanced muscle strength. You might even rig a bungee cord from the top of your helmet to the top of the cockpit. On long missions this helps hold the head up and eases stresses on the neck muscles. After the mission you would need to know how to hold the head correctly balanced on the shoulders to establish balanced muscle strength. Balanced muscle strength would ensure proper alignment and maximize recovery. It would ensure the head wouldn't lean too far this or that way and injure the nerve roots in its altered state. This way you wouldn't have to consider the neck, back, shoulder pain, numbness, tingling or early retirement as part of the price you pay to protect a way of life.

In this example:

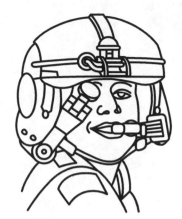

**Image 1.10**
**Helicopter pilot with helmet.**

1) **The degree of departure from the natural body position seems more severe in the Asian women;**
2) **The rationale is different;**
3) **The neck is the body part affected in both examples.**

Recovery could be complete for either one if symmetry and balance were considered in the recovery process.

**Nature vs. Culture**

These are a few examples and there are many more. The point being made is that the body can be altered by cultural-postural habits and artifacts. The impact of habit is highly significant. Bodies were created to be used in a certain manner. They are machines that, when used according to manufacturer's specifications, will function properly and maintain their proper form for life. Get yourself used to the natural, balanced way of standing as will be explained. Your body will maintain its proper form, even tone and function, without exercise. It will do it with no more effort than you now habitually exert with your unnatural, uncentered, unbalanced, asymmetrical way of standing or walking.

Let me explain how this works. There are all the associated familiar sayings that influence us to behave and position ourselves in certain ways: get dressed up, put on some dress shoes, stand at attention, sit up straight, stand up straight with your chin up, chest out and stomach in, show some respect, show some confidence, have some pride in yourself, put some bounce in your step, etc. When these behaviors and positions become habitual, they are maintained long enough, repeated often enough, or both, for the body's form to be altered. These alterations are then commonly thought of as poor posture or the aging process.

If you're involved in an occupation where you're required to stand with the knees locked back, adopt an unnatural gait, sit up straight at attention due to protocol (such as the military), do so. If you must be subject to severe activity/ equipment loads, by all means do so. Whether it's done to obtain a livelihood or defend a livelihood. The reasons for placing yourself in positions that, if maintained, can alter your physical form may be desirable and necessary. Just remember the correct way to stand, sit and walk that you'll learn in this book. Then, when you're off work, return to them as soon, as often, and as long as possible. You will maximize recovery and return to work in peak condition in minimal time. You will achieve maximum longevity.

If you must sit in a certain manner in a straight chair to show respect or assume a persona in a circumstance, do so. When you get the chance, recline, recline, recline. If you feel you must wear those high-heeled pointy shoes, do so. If you must wear headgear and sustain activity loads that make your neck sore and alter your balanced muscle strength, do so. If you want to amplify a posture to look attractive, confident, command respect, show respect or look respectable, do so. If you assume a position to attain goodness or look good, to obtain enlightenment or to look enlightened, that's fine. An unbalanced position may just be a habit you picked up somewhere, somehow without realizing it. But unlike the nose in front of your face or the culture you're immersed in, be aware of them. Habits can potentially alter your physical form. Be aware of what they are doing to your body. Make the body altering positions you assume and/or artifacts you use, the activity of the moment. Make the natural, balanced body positioning you will learn in this book the habit of your real life. Your body will thank you for it with a properly proportioned, evenly toned appearance. You will achieve maximum performance and longevity for your entire life.

Without exercise.

# Chapter One
# Why Posture Is Not Perfect
## Part Two:
## Nuts, Bolts and Behavior of the Body

This chapter will complete the process of explaining the dynamics of posture. It will describe the reactions caused inside the body by positional habits themselves and positional habits associated with artifacts.

It's difficult to realistically model biological forms, but it's necessary to fully understand what's going on in the human body we're immersed in. In this chapter, I'll get inside the body – under the skin, so to speak. Through comparison, I'll show how these habits affect the actual nuts, bolts and mechanical behavior of the body. I'll compare a spring to a body. Much of the focus will be on the spine, since that is the body part most noticeably affected. It's also the body part that most resembles a spring and is therefore easiest to associate with a spring. But keep in mind, many joints of the body are affected at the same time, by the same definitions and laws of nature. Those equally affected would include the pelvis, hips, knees and foot joints.

This comparison will give a step-by-step explanation of what the spring and body are, what they do and why they do it. It will give those of you not familiar with anatomy and its seeming complexity something you can identify with and understand in the everyday world. You'll also learn a little about spring mechanics.

There are a few things you should know before I get started.

In this comparison some difficulties arose because a spring is missing one comparable part. The spring and body each have a comparable axis or midline. The spring has coils and the body has comparable bones or vertebra. And here is the difficulty. The spring does not have anything surrounding its coils comparable to the skin and all that soft stuff that a body has surrounding its bones. So, for purposes of this comparison, the spring will have to have an imaginary body. The coils will have to have an imaginary skin with soft stuff underneath that surrounds them. It won't invalidate the comparison. The spring's coils would still behave the same with flesh and skin covering them. The flesh and skin would behave like the flesh and skin covering the body if the spring had them. You'll just have to have a little imagination.

Springs and bodies have some other differences I'll touch on as I go along.

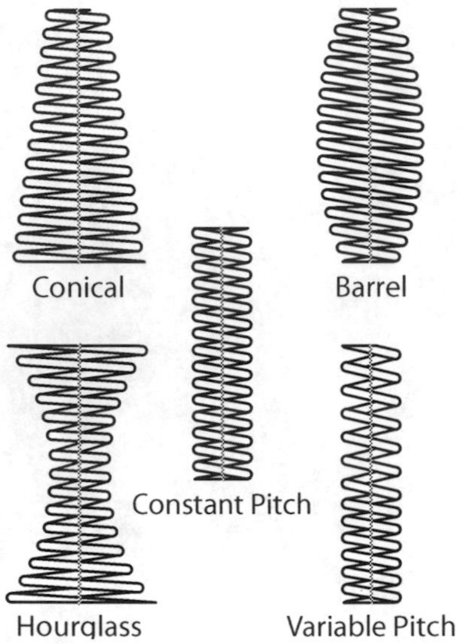

The descriptions of the spring will be of a general nature. This is because springs can come with a widely varied number of coils and configurations. They can be tall, short, narrow, wide or whatever shape with constant or variable pitch. Human bodies have a set number of vertebrae or bones. They too can be tall, short, narrow, wide or whatever shape and have different variations of pitch. But, basic configuration is more limited. Characteristics and behaviors, in either case, remain the same. So there will be no names or numbers for the various coils. Various bones and vertebrae will be named and numbered for more detailed understanding.

In the process of preparing for this comparison, I found there are many definitions for one and the same characteristic or behavior in the spring. It's the same with the body. This gave me many definitions from both structures for a single characteristic or behavior that is common to both. The potential for confusion is great. So in the process of this comparison, one, at most two, suitable terms will be chosen that will apply to the same characteristic or behavior as it occurs in both. It will clearly define the concept to ensure understanding and make it easy to cross reference. It will keep you from getting confused with a lot of different names for the same thing. Definitions that aren't technical, complicated, or unfamiliar to most will be used. It will make it easier in case you're not a spring engineer, anatomist (specialist in body structure) or physiologist (specialist in body function).

Conical

Barrel

Constant Pitch

Hourglass

Variable Pitch

**Image 2.01**

**A spring can have any configuration, in other words, number, shape, spacing, thickness and angle of coils. The engineering characteristics and mechanical behavior remain the same.**

Another thing you should be aware of so this comparison is clearly understandable. A body has an obvious front (anterior), back (posterior) and sides. A spring does not. Its directional orientation is dictated by the surrounding structure. A spring, without a directional point of reference, could be seen as facing any which way whatsoever. Depending on the notion of the observer it could be seen as facing forward, back, side to side or diagonal. Can't have that. In this explanation, the direction of the cause and effect behaviors in spring or spine are important. You'll need to picture the springs or body parts having an anterior, posterior and sides. The springs will have the same directional orientation as the figures they are being immediately compared to. In this comparison all springs and figures will face either to the left, front or the back.

Springs are fundamental mechanical components that form the basis for many mechanical systems, natural or engineered. The engineering characteristics and mechanical behavior of compression springs have been extensively studied, tested and documented. These characteristics and behaviors are the same in the spine and body. Therefore, by comparing the engineering characteristics and mechanical behavior of a spring to a spine and body, we can better understand the spine and body's engineering characteristics and mechanical behavior. The body is generally much more flexible and mobile than a spring but it has its limits, and it too is ultimately affected by the same dynamics and laws of nature.

The spring is usually regarded as a fairly simple machine. The body is usually regarded as a complex machine. Neither consideration about either is totally true. Both have basic characteristics and behaviors that can be analyzed to the point of high complexity. The basics are all you need to know to have Perfect Posture. Once I've got basics explained, I'll quickly show how complicated it can get. Then, if you're of a mind to delve further into such things, you can.

Similar engineering characteristics will be considered first. These characteristics are of an all or nothing type of association. If even one characteristic is out of shape or unbalanced, it will distort all the others to the same degree and distort the whole structure.

## Engineering Characteristics

### The central axis

The first of the characteristics that a spring and body share is a point or line, within a circle of physical symmetry, called an "axis." An axis is defined as a central line bisecting a body, form, or the like, in relation to which symmetry is determined.

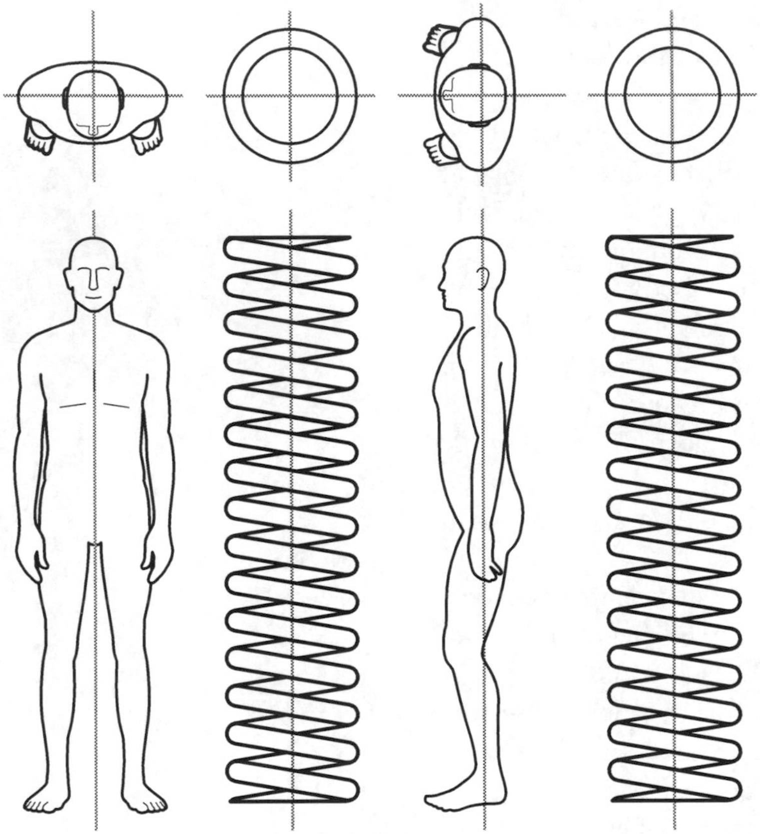

In the spring, the location of the axis and how the coils are symmetrically positioned around it is extensively considered, studied and documented by spring engineers. It's the midline of the spring running from end to end. In the spring, this midline is variously called, but not limited to, the "central axis of the frame," "central axis," "helix axis," "line of gravity" or "meridian."

In the body, the equivalent concept of the axis, its location and how the body is symmetrically positioned around it is not as extensively considered, studied, or documented.

What is needed in the case of the body, then, is to clearly identify where this midline bisects the body and how to symmetrically position the body around it. Image 2.02 illustrates the properly positioned central axis of a spring and body. I will give step-by-step instructions on exactly how to position the body, so it surrounds the axis symmetrically, in

**Image 2.02**
**Properly positioned central axis, side to side, front to back and top to bottom.**

the next chapter.

A single term for a clear definition is also needed. I'll use the term "central axis" or "axis" for defining the "midline in relation to which symmetry is determined" in reference to both spring and body.

## The axial load

Another important engineering characteristics common to a spring and body is that each is designed to have a weight or force exerted upon it.

The position and dynamics of the weight or force exerted on the spring is extensively considered, studied and measured. It can be just about anything from boxcars to flashlight batteries. It can be static or cyclic. It is variously defined as, but not limited to, its "load," "load components," "surface forces," or "body forces." With accurate positioning, the load is evenly balanced above, below and the length of the spring's central axis. When in this balanced position, it is called an "axial load." Tension, or stress level, will be equal at opposite points on each side of the axis on the plane of the load. A balanced or "axial load" is essential for a properly proportioned and evenly toned spring. [Image 2.03]

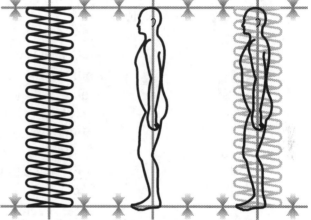

Image 2.03
The load must be evenly balanced, be it spring or body, for a straight and evenly toned structure.

The position and dynamics of this weight or force exerted on the body is not as extensively considered, studied or measured. In the case of the body, this weight or force is gravity. Gravity's effects can also be static or cyclic. (Jump off your porch to prove this.) It's variously defined as, but not limited to, "effects of gravity," "pull of gravity," "gravitational force," or "Gs." How to position gravity evenly, balanced upon the body above, below and the length of the body's central axis will be shown. A balanced or "axial gravitational force" is essential for a properly proportioned, and evenly toned body.

I'll use the term "axial load" for defining the "characteristic of having a weight, force or gravity in the case of the body, evenly balanced above, below and the length of the central axis" of spring and body.

## Balancing stresses, tension or tone

When the push of a point or object up is equal to the pull of a load or gravity down on that point or object, a state of equilibrium exists. The point or object between these two forces will not move up or down. The strength of this pushing up and pulling down is the tone, tension or stress level on the point or object in between. Let me explain how this works. If you hold a 10 pound weight steady in your hand, the push of your hand up would be 10 pounds. The pull of the load/gravity down would be 10 pounds. If you increased the weight to 20 pounds, the tone, tension or stress level on the hand will have doubled. It would triple for 30 pounds and so on. [Image 2.04]

In any structure, this push up-pull down effect will have a balanced tone, tension or stress level on either side of the arrangement's axis. If not, it will bend, fall over or collapse. In an evenly balanced spring or body, stresses, tension or tone will be equal above and below at opposite points, front to back and side to side, from top to bottom for the length of the axis. If this is not so, the spring or body will not be properly proportioned and evenly toned. It will be in the process of bending, falling over, bulging or collapsing.

I'll use the terms "stresses, tension or tone" inter-changeably for defining the "strength at which a point or object is being pushed up by the force of a spring or body, and, at the same time, pulled down by the force of its load or gravity" in reference to both spring and body.

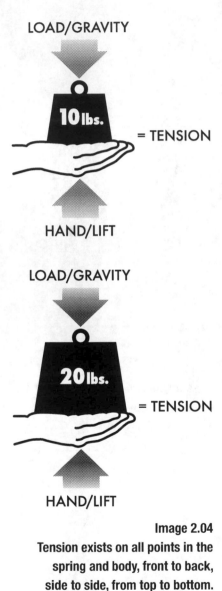

**Image 2.04**

Tension exists on all points in the spring and body, front to back, side to side, from top to bottom.

## Pitch and angle

The spring is created with coils meant to function at a certain distance from each other. In spring terminology, the distance from the middle of one coil to the middle of the next is called "pitch." [Image 2.05] Angle would be the degree of slant between any two coils for one measure of pitch. The pitch and angle of the coils will vary with load fluctuations. They should vary according to the creator's specifications for intended use in a particular, predetermined relation to each other.

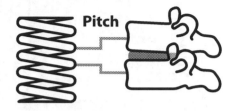

**Image 2.05**
**Pitch of balanced spring and vertebras.**

Your body is created with bones meant to function at a certain distance from each other. I haven't found a definition in human terminology for the distance from the middle of one vertebra to the middle of the next. So I'll use a concept and definition from spring terminology interchangeably for the human model. In this comparison, "pitch" will refer to the distance between the middle of the body of one vertebra to the middle of the body of the next vertebra. [Image 2.05] "Angle" will be the degree of slant between any two bodies of vertebra for one measure of pitch. [Image 2.06] The pitch and angle of the vertebras will vary with load fluctuations. They should vary according to the Creator's specifications for intended use and in a particular predetermined relation to each other. Remember that the joints of the pelvis, hip, knee and foot are affected at the same time, in the same way, by the same definitions, etc.

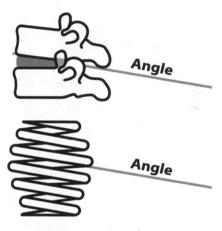

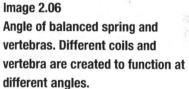

**Image 2.06**
**Angle of balanced spring and vertebras. Different coils and vertebra are created to function at different angles.**

Note: In this comparison, the meaning of the word "pitch" may be different from what you are used to. It doesn't mean slope or slant of something such as a roof or the ground. Don't get confused.

## Spaces

The spring is created with spaces between the coils meant to function in certain shapes. In spring technology, oddly enough, these spaces are called "spaces between the coils." The shape of the spaces between coils will vary

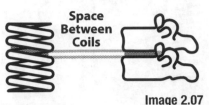

**Image 2.07**
Space between the coils and vertebras will vary.

with load fluctuations, but they should vary according to the creator's specifications for intended use and in a particular predetermined relation to each other.

The body is created with spaces between the bones meant to function in certain shapes. In the body these spaces, not so oddly it seems, are called "joints," "spinal disks," "intravertebral disks," or simply "disks." [Image 2.07]

The shape of the spaces between vertebras will vary with load fluctuations, but they should vary according to the Creator's specifications for intended use and in a particular predetermined relation to each other.

In this comparison I'll use the term "spaces" to define "the area between coils in the spring" and "disks" to define "the area between vertebrae in the body."

You now know the engineering characteristics necessary to understand Perfect Posture. These characteristics are common to all properly proportioned, balanced and evenly toned springs and bodies.

You now know the definitions we will be using to refer to these individual, shared characteristics.

## Summary of Engineering Characteristics for Spring and Spine

The properly proportioned, balanced and evenly toned spring or body will always have a bisecting line running from end to end called an axis. The coils or body will always be symmetrically positioned around it. Each will carry a weight or force that will be evenly balanced upon it, called an axial load. Tension or stresses will be equal at opposite points above and below, front to back and side to side, from top to bottom, for the length of the axis. Each will have coils or vertebras that are created to be at a certain pitch or distance from each other. Each will be created to have a certain angle between these coils and vertebras. Each will have spaces between the coils or vertebras. The pitch, angle and shape of the spaces will vary with load fluctuations, but they will vary in a particular, predetermined relation to each other.

These engineering characteristics apply to all proportioned, balanced and evenly toned variable stress compression springs and bodies, no matter the shape or configuration. It doesn't matter whether it/he/she is tall, short, narrow or wide,

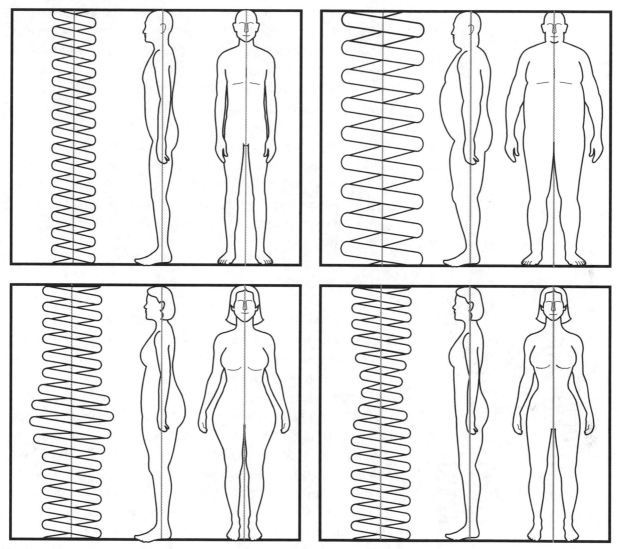

It doesn't matter whether it/he/she is hourglass, barrel, pear shaped, long lower configuration or legs, short lower configuration or legs, pregnant or otherwise. It doesn't matter whether the ends are round or flat. [Image 2.08]

**Image 2.08**
**Characteristics remain the same no matter what the shape is.**

## MECHANICAL BEHAVIORS

### The Origin of Crooked Springs and Bodies

I'll now compare mechanical behaviors of the spring to their equivalent behaviors in the body. Examination will show that the spring and body exhibit the same behaviors when the same conditions are applied. The condition of concern in this comparison is an unbalanced, non-axial or tilted load. This is because the ultimate origin of a warped spring, or imperfect posture, is a tilted load. The spring and body's response to tilt is the behavior of concern. A tilting of the load, in spring or body, anywhere along the length of the axis, causes tension to become unbalanced and the axis to warp or bend. The surrounding form of the spring or body then follows the bend of the axis and becomes shaped in the same contours. It can have many causes in either the spring or the body.

### Tilt and the spring

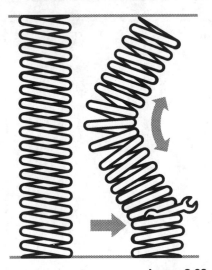

**Image 2.09**
**A monkey wrench into the works.**

In the spring, the reasons for a tilted load are limitless. The reasons for the severity of the tilt are limitless. The tilt can occur at the top, bottom or anywhere in between. It can be due to one or a combination of reasons. It could be due to a mechanical accident such as a broken upper flange or mount. It could be due to a flaw in the material the spring is made from. It could be a loose piece of the surrounding structure becoming lodged in the coils, tilting it somewhere along its length. It could be a worker's tool falling between a pair of coils. It could even be a combination of all of these. If the shift or tilt is brief, it will not cause extensive alteration in the spring's structure. If the shift or tilt is severe, prolonged, repetitive or all three, it may surpass what is called the elastic limit. "Elastic limit" is the maximum stress to which a material may be subjected without causing permanent structural changes. If these permanent changes occur they are called "plastic deformation", or "permanent set." The spring will never resume its previous shape even if recentered permanently. [Image 2.09]

### Tilt and the body

In the body, the reasons for a tilted load are limitless. The reasons for the severity of the tilt are limitless. The tilt can occur at the top, the bottom or anywhere in between. It can be due to one or a combination of reasons. It could be due to a mechanical artifact such as a heavy helmet. It could be a flaw in the material the body is made from. It could be a postural habit like a pair of locked knees tilting the body forward along its length. It could be a fashion artifact like high heels worn often. It could even be a combination of all of these. If the shift or tilt is brief, it will not cause extensive alteration in the body's structure. If the shift or tilt is severe, prolonged, repetitive or all three, it may surpass the point of what is called the ability to recover. If these changes are irreversible they are called "permanent disability" or "debility." But, the body is much more flexible than a metal spring. A body can heal and is capable of adjustments with centering or Perfect Posturing almost no matter how severe, prolonged or repetitive the tilt. The spring cannot. The body has a much greater ability to resume its previous shape if re-centering becomes a habit.

In the body, the vast majority of the time the load is tilted, locking the knees back is the predominant cause. The effects can be corrected the vast majority of the time. The focus of this book is on this cause and the correction of its effects.

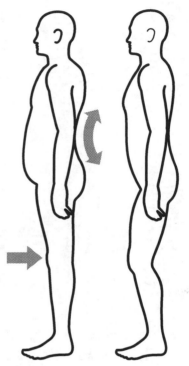

**Image 2.10**
**Locked knees throw a monkey wrench into the body's natural balance.**

### The General Response to Tilt

In the spring or body, if there is a balanced or axial load upon the axis, tension will be equal at corresponding opposite points on the plane of the load. The axis will remain straight and symmetrically positioned. A perpendicular plane placed anywhere on the length of the axis will have equal tension above and below it, at corresponding opposite points on that

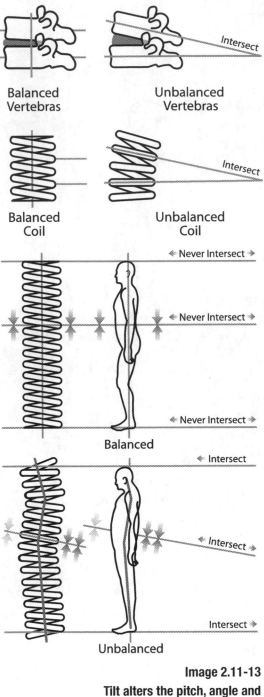

Balanced
Vertebras

Unbalanced
Vertebras

Intersect

Balanced
Coil

Unbalanced
Coil

Never Intersect

Never Intersect

Never Intersect

Balanced

Intersect

Intersect

Intersect

Unbalanced

**Image 2.11-13**

**Tilt alters the pitch, angle and
spacing of coils and vertebras.**

plane. The plane will never tilt, like an unbalanced teeter-totter, and intersect with the horizontal line of the axial load. It always will remain parallel to the plane of the axial load. Thus, when the load is balanced, the correct pitch of all the spring's coils and the spine's vertebrae will be maintained. The correct space between all the coils and vertebra will also be maintained. Spring, spine and body will maintain their proper proportion, even tone and optimum performance.

If this is not so, tensions become unbalanced. All the coils, vertebrae and spaces are altered to some degree along the entire length of the structure. It does not affect only the coils or vertebrae in the immediate area of the occurrence.

The object of the preceding explanation and illustration is to clarify the important fact that all of the individual coils in a spring work mechanically as single units. At the same time, they are part of a larger structure and also function within that context. If just one individual coil is effected or tilted anywhere along the spring, the entire structure is affected, top to bottom.

It also must be understood that all of the individual body parts, head, vertebrae, legs, and feet, also work mechanically as single units. At the same time, they too are part of the larger structure and also function within that context. If just one part is effected or tilted anywhere along the body, the entire structure is affected top to bottom.

An expression to reinforce this concept: There must be mutual/equal weight on all sides of the spring and spine at each level, or the integrity of the whole is lost. In other words, if one part fails, the entire structure fails or is at least compromised to some degree.

## A DETAILED EXAMINATION OF
## THE RESPONSE TILT

### Mechanical Failure and Buckle in the Spring

In a load-bearing spring with a length greater than four times the spring diameter, if the load is tilted off the axis, structures undergo a relatively large instantaneous change. The effect of this large instantaneous change is to cause a bulge, bend or bow in the axis and, therefore, in the entire structure of the spring. In spring terminology, this is variously called, but not limited to, "buckling, "deformation," "bucking," or even "flying out sideways." The initial buckle will occur in the direction of the tilt. Typically, the effect occurs midway between the point of tilt and the other end of the structure. Typically, the buckle comes to an apex or peak at a point midway between two particular coils. [Image 2.14]

This has other effects on the spring not confined to the immediate area of the buckle. On the tilted or posterior side of the spring diameter, pitch is decreased and tension is increased. Pitch decreases and tension increases to maximum at the posterior apex. On the non-tilted, front or anterior side of the spring diameter, pitch is increased and tension is decreased (Remember, it's facing left.) Pitch increases and tension decreases to minimum at the anterior apex. The effects radiate out, lessening from the apex of the buckle.

This example only will use a spring tilted about one fourth up its length from the bottom. This is to emphasize the idea that it's the knee that is commonly the point of weight shift or tilt in the body. A box wrench lodged in the coils at the equivalent level will represent locking the knees back. A spring structure tilted at the bottom will be used in the remainder of the book. This will keep it basic for simplicity of understanding and ease of illustration. The same basic cause and effect principles apply with tilt, no matter where it occurs on the spring.

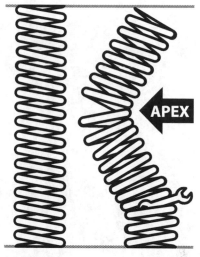

**Image 2.14**
**A monkey wrench in the posture of the spring at the comparative knee level.**

## Locking the Knees and Lordosis in the Body

In a load-bearing body, with a length greater than four times the body diameter, if an axial load is tilted off of the axis, by locking the knees back, structures undergo a relatively large, instantaneous change. The effect of this large instantaneous change is to cause a bulge, bend or bow in the spine and, therefore, in the entire structure of the body. In human terminology, this is called "Lordosis," "deformation," "deviation," or even, "bending over backwards." The initial bulge will occur in the direction of the tilt. Typically, the effect occurs midway between the point of tilt and the other end of the structure. Ordinarily, the Lordosis comes to an apex or peak at a point midway between two central vertebras. The common point of tilt in humans is at the knee, when it is locked to the rear rather than kept in a *slightly* bent position. This immediately causes the spine, at the lumbar vertebras 1 through 5 and the sacrum, to bulge forward. The apex of this bulge in humans is usually at the disk between the L3 and L4 vertebras. This translates to the "bellybutton-level spine." The pelvis tips to the front at the same time, the effects of which will be explained in Chapter Two. [Image 2.15]

This has other effects on the body, most notably but not confined to the immediate area of the bulge. On the *posterior* side of the spinal diameter, pitch is decreased and tension is increased. Pitch decreases and tension increases to maximum at the posterior apex. On the anterior side of the spinal diameter pitch is increased and tension is decreased. Pitch increases and tension decreases to minimum at the anterior apex. The effects radiate out, lessening from the apex or middle of the bulge.

I will use the term **buckle** to define the "large instantaneous change, or bulge, with a tilt of the axial load" in reference to both spring and body. **Apex** will define "the head, summit or peak of the buckle at a point midway between two central coils or vertebras in the spring or spine."

Buckle occurs in all compression springs and all bodies if the load is unbalanced along the axis: Top, bottom, or

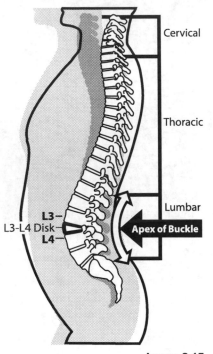

**Image 2.15**
**The apex of the buckle at the L3 - L4 disk.**

anywhere in between. No matter the shape or configuration. It doesn't matter whether it/he/she is tall, short, narrow or wide,

It doesn't matter whether it/he/she is hourglass, barrel, pear shaped, long lower configuration or legs, short lower configuration or legs, pregnant or otherwise. It doesn't matter whether the ends are round or flat. If the load is unbalanced, buckle will occur.

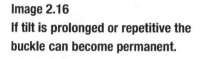

**Image 2.16**
**If tilt is prolonged or repetitive the buckle can become permanent.**

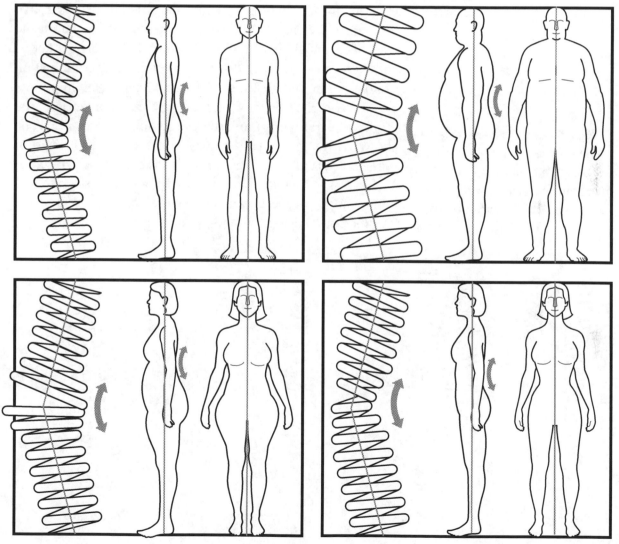

## Time + Buckle = Creep

### Creep and the spring

In the spring, after the large instantaneous buckling, there follows a slower, time-dependent change that can differ in form due to numerous variables. In the technical jargon of spring engineers, this time-dependent change is variously called, but not limited to, "creep," "drift," or "deflection." Creep occurs in two distinct types though never in complete isolation from each other. There is the type that occurs **above** the apex of the buckle. There is the type that occurs **below** the apex of the buckle. You might see a combination of 30% above and 70% below the apex creep. You might see a combination of 30% below and 70% above the apex creep. You might see a 50-50 combination. I will not address a combination of the two in illustration. A rendering of combinations will not be shown as it's impossible to clearly depict the full range of potential variables. I'll try to show as pure an example of each type as possible. That way, when one of those countless combinations of these two is encountered, you'll realize it's not that complicated - it's just some combination of the two.

**Image 2.17**

**From the left: a perfectly balanced spring, a tilted spring with the initial buckle, a spring illustrating time-dependent creep above the buckle, a spring illustrating time-dependent creep below the buckle.**

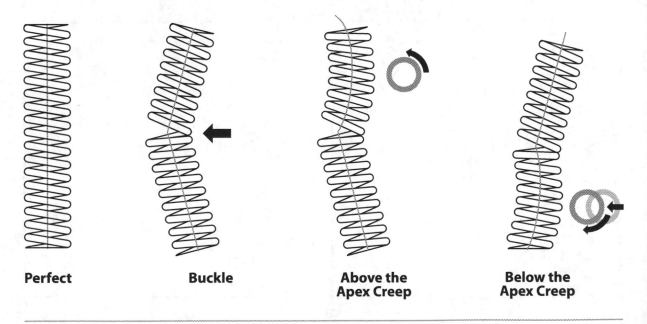

**Perfect**     **Buckle**     **Above the Apex Creep**     **Below the Apex Creep**

## Dynamics of creep in the spring

Analysis shows that the distribution of tension becomes more uniform over the cross sections of the coils after creep has occurred. It might be said creep is nature's way of sharing all that tension concentrated in the backside of the buckle with the rest of the spring. It could be compared to water finding a common level and so on.

This is how it works in **above**-the-buckle creep. Pitch increases in the backside of the coils and decreases in the front – mostly above the apex. As a result, tension is decreased in back and increased in front. Thus, tension is more uniform on both sides of the structure, front and back. The buckle shares the tension with the coils above.

In **below**-the-buckle creep, pitch increases in the backside of the coils and decreases in front – mostly below the apex. As a result, tension is decreased in the backside of the coils and increased in front. Thus tension is more uniform on both sides of the structure, front and back. The buckle shares the tension with the coils below.

Note the use of the word **mostly** in reference to above- and below-the-apex creep. What affects one part of the spring affects the rest of the structure. There is no such thing as pure above- or pure below-the-apex of the-buckle-creep. They exist as a basic idea or possibility to help you understand what you are seeing when they are mixed together in different combinations. These effects ripple out from the affected area to the entire spring. By understanding the basics, you can understand the infinite combinations that happen with them.

To varying degrees and form, creep occurs in all compression springs if the load is tilted off center and the coils are buckled for extended periods, repeatedly or both. The more unbalanced the load, the more the buckle. The more time spent buckled, the more the creep.

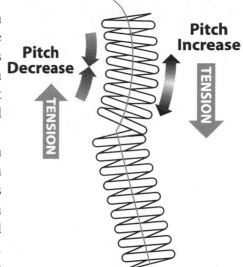

**Above the Buckle Creep**

Image 2.18 & 2.19
Buckle declines as stress distribution becomes more uniform over cross sections after creep has occurred.

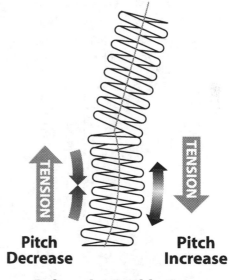

**Below the Buckle Creep**

## Deformity and the body

Similarly, in the body, after a large instantaneous buckling, there follows a slower, time-dependent change that can differ in form due to numerous variables. In the technical jargon of health professionals, this time-dependent change is variously called, but not limited to, "deformity," "kyphosis," "Dowagers hump," or "hypolordosis." In common language, it might be called "hunchback," "slumping shoulders," "droop," "slouch," "swayback," "flat *ss," "aging process," "gettin' old," "poor posture," or even "a creep." (We could go on for a long time. There are lots and lots of them).

Similar to the spring's creep, deformity occurs in two distinct types though never in complete isolation from each other. There is the type that occurs **above** the apex of the buckle. There is the type that occurs **below** the apex of the buckle. You might be, or see, a 30% above- and 70% below-this-level creep. You might be, or see, a 30% below- and 70% above-this-level creep. You might be, or see, a 50-50 combination. I will not address combinations of the two in illustration. A rendering of combinations will not be shown as it's impossible to clearly depict the full range of potential variables. I'll try to show as pure an example as possible of each type. That way, when one of those countless combinations is encountered, you'll realize it's really not that complicated. It's just some combination of the two.

**Image 2.20**
**Shaded profile is where perfect posture should be. The outline shows the movement of the spine and body with buckle and creep.**

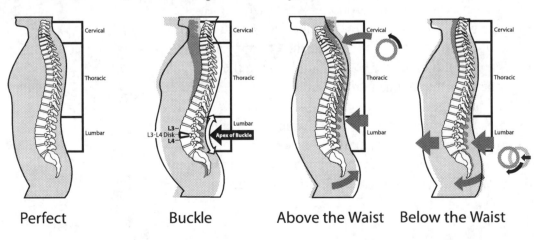

Perfect          Buckle          Above the Waist          Below the Waist

## Dynamics of deformity in the body

As in the spring, analysis shows that the distribution of tension becomes more uniform over the cross sections of the vertebras after deformity has occurred. It might be said, deformity is nature's way of sharing all that tension concentrated in the back side of the buckle with the rest of the spine. It could be compared to water finding a common level, and so on.

This is how it works in **above**-the-buckle or waist deformity. Pitch increases on the backside of the vertebrae and decreases in the front – mostly above the apex. As a result, tension is decreased in back and increased in front. Thus, tension is more uniform on both sides of the structure, front and back. The buckle shares the tension with the vertebrae above.

In **below**-the-buckle or waist deformity, pitch increases in the backside of the vertebrae mostly below the apex, or L3 and L4 disks and decreases in front. As a result, tension has decreased in the back and increased in front. Thus, tension is more uniform on both sides of the structure, front and back. The buckle shares the tension with the vertebrae below.

Note the use of the word **mostly** in reference to above- or below-the-apex deformity. What affects one part of the spine affects the rest of the structure. There is no such thing as pure above or pure below the apex deformity. They exist

Image 2.21
**Shaded profile represents balanced body and spring.**
**A. Outline overlay represents buckled body and spring.**
**B. Outlined overlay represents above the apex deformity or creep in the body and spring.**
**C. Outlined overlay represents below the apex deformity or creep in the body and spring.**

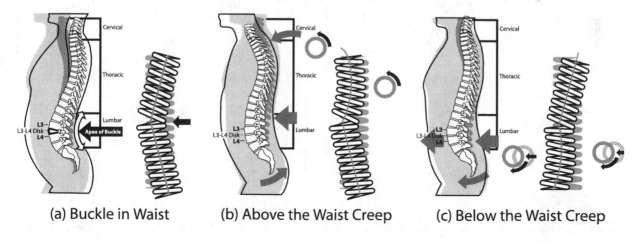

(a) Buckle in Waist    (b) Above the Waist Creep    (c) Below the Waist Creep

Thin man with above the waist creep. Thick man with above the waist creep. Pear shaped woman with below the waist creep and hourglass shaped woman with below the waist creep. Note how the shape of the spring's ax'es have the same contours as the bodies.

as a basic idea or possibility to help you understand what you are seeing when they are mixed together in different combinations. These effects ripple out from the affected area to the entire spine. No two spines, springs or ripples behave exactly the same, but they do have basic characteristics in common. By understanding the basics, you can understand the infinite combinations that happen with them.

To varying degrees and shape, a deformity occurs in all bodies if the load is tilted off center and the axis is buckled for extended periods, repeatedly, or both. The more unbalanced,

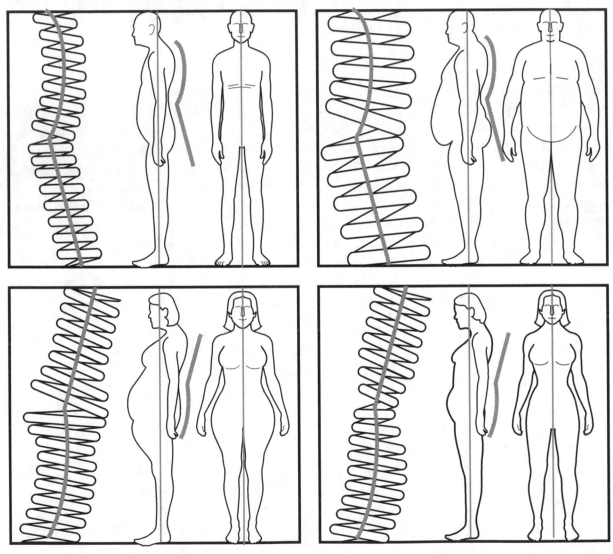

the more the buckle. The more time spent buckled, the more the deformity.

Creep seems to have a memorable ring to it. I'll use the term "creep" for defining the "slower, time dependent change that is varied following buckling" in reference to both spring and body.

Creep occurs in all compression springs and bodies if the load is unbalanced and the coils or vertebrae are buckled for sufficient amount of time, no matter the shape or configuration. [Image 2.27] It doesn't matter whether it/he/she is tall, short, narrow or wide. It doesn't matter whether it/he/she is hourglass, barrel, pear shaped, long lower configuration or legs, short lower configuration or legs, pregnant or otherwise. It doesn't matter whether the ends are round or flat.

## BASICS WILL DO

### Complicating the Spring

You now know the basics. Any more detail is unnecessary. The following is a sample of what the details would involve if you care to go further.

The reasons buckle and creep can take many different forms and periods of time are few and easy to understand. It's when you mix them together in different quantities that things get complicated.

In the spring, it basically boils down to three contributing factors.

The first is the material from which the spring is made, the strength of its chemical composition. The stuff it's made of (shear modulus), $G$; in effect – its strength and resistance to change (elastic limit), $E$.

Second is the basic shape of the spring: height, width, thickness of the coils, spacing between the coils, or even segmented structures with variously pitched, angled and spaced coils (coil slenderness ratio), $n$.

Third are the unique circumstances of the particular

spring's environment – in other words, the degree of tilt and the amount of time tilted (deflection), δ.

But, the basic principles are the same whether the spring is made from titanium or pig iron. The same no matter what the configuration is. To varying degrees, buckling followed by creep occurs in all compression springs, with a length greater than four times the spring diameter if the load is off center. The more the tilt, the more the buckle, the more time buckled, the more the creep.

I could discuss how load-per-unit deflection (spring rate), $k$, can be made to vary widely:

**Image 2.23**
**Load Per Unit Formula**

$$k = \frac{P}{\delta} = \frac{G}{8}\frac{d^4}{D^3 n} = \frac{E}{16(1+v)}\frac{d^4}{D^3 n}$$

Where "δ" is the deflection, **G** is the shear modulus and **v** is Poisson's ratio.

But I won't.

So none of the stuff below will be discussed, explained or expanded (and believe me, this is just scratching the surface).

**Image 2.24**
**Strain Percent Graph**

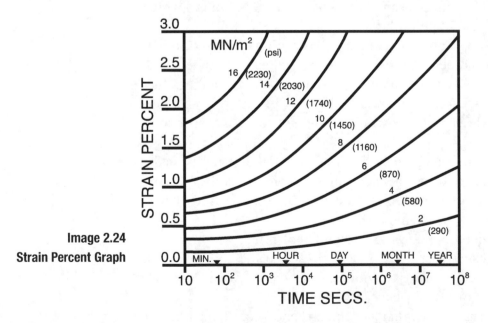

We will deal with the basics:

**a) Tilt** of the axial load – possible reasons in the spring are too numerous to consider;

**b)** Initial **buckle**. Typically midway between the point of tilt and the end of the structure;

**c)** The inevitable time-dependent **creep** occurring in two basic types.

There will be none of the countless equations and graphs for combinations of variables in this book. Keep it simple and basic. Tilt happens. When it happens buckle results. Creep follows if the tilt and buckle is prolonged, repetitive or both – period. If you wish to go further, you'll have to do it on your own.

If all of these details interests you, contact the *Spring Manufacturers Institute*. They're looking for the next generation of spring engineers.

## Complicating the Body

It's the same with a weight-bearing spine and body. Things can get complicated. Buckle, and then creep, can take many forms and periods of time to occur. But, you know all you need to so that the rest of the book can be followed with an understanding of what you are doing and why. The reasons for the "how to get it" and "how to keep it section" should be clear.

In the human, it also boils down to three comparable factors, much the same as in the spring. These factors are easy to understand individually, but when mixed together in different quantities can make the subject seem complicated and intimidating.

The first is the material the individual is made of, the strength of the individual's chemical composition. This includes the inherited endowment (genetics), plus health of the individual (health index). In other words, how strong the body is to begin with and how well it's been taken care of. If an individual is born strong, eats a healthy diet, and exercises, the body's material composition would be chemically stronger and more resistant to change (alteration rate).

Second is basic shape of the body: tall, short, thick, or thin. Tall and thin is more susceptible to gravity's effects than short and thick. Buckle and creep is also easier to see when you're tall and thin (slenderness ratio).

Third are the unique circumstances of the individual's environment. In other words, the degree of tilt (poor posture ratio) and amount of time spent tilted. Or, you could say the activities of daily living (ADL).

I could also dwell long and hard on cultural evolution and habits — things like how and why they evolve. But, that's a subject that could fill another book, so I won't do that either. *But, why do people stand with the knees locked back?*

I'm sure I could come up with some decent-looking equations and graphs to rival spring mechanics for countless combinations of variables in the comparison. Covering any, mathematically or graphically, is much beyond the necessary scope of this book. It's probably much beyond your thirst for knowledge on the subject. It's absolutely beyond mine. So I won't.

No more condensed or distilled definitions.

This book will cover the basics only:

**a) Tilt** of the axial load and the most common cause: locking the knees back.

**b)** The instantaneous **buckle** of the spine at the waist level with pelvic tilt.

**c)** The time-dependent **creep** that follows.

These are simple, easy-to-understand principles of tilt, buckle, and creep. All the virtuous, mannerly, respectful, idealistic intentions will have little effect. Exercise and proper nutrition will have little more. Fundamental dynamics, though subject to infinite variables, accepted as fact in spring engineering circles and equally applicable to the spine and body. You can see why I wanted to keep this simple. If you wish to delve into complexities, feel free.

## A Side-by-Side Summary and Description of Tilt, Buckle, and Creep's Effect in the Spring and Body

### Tilt and buckle in the spring and body

When the axial load is tilted to the front, a spring and spine undergo the relatively large instantaneous change. Their axis is buckled toward the front along with the coils of the spring and spine of the body. On the backside of the spring's coils and spine's vertebras pitch is decreased and tension is increased. On the front side, pitch is increased and tension is decreased. In the spring, this is comparative to a buckled back, compressed spinal disks on the rear side of the lumbar backbone, forward tipped pelvis, stretch weakened soft-bulging abdomen and the start of low back problems we see so much. In the body, this is the actual buckle of the back, compressed spinal disks on the rear side of the lumbar backbone, forward tipped pelvis, stretch weakened soft-bulging abdomen and the start of low back problems we see so often.

**Image 2.25**
**Shaded profiles are balanced spring and body. If you take a slinky™ and buckle it, the coils on the front of the apex are flaccid. This is the same effect occurring with the spine and abdomen.**

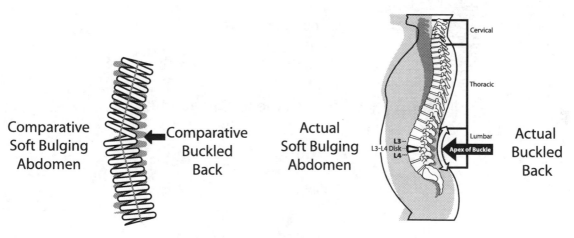

Comparative Soft Bulging Abdomen ← Comparative Buckled Back

Actual Soft Bulging Abdomen

Cervical

Thoracic

Lumbar

L3
L3-L4 Disk
L4

**Apex of Buckle**

Actual Buckled Back

## Buckle in the Spring and Body

### Creep above the buckle

Creep occurring above the buckle in the spring is comparable to creep above the L 3- 4 vertebral disk or belly button level spine in the body. The coils of the spring and vertebra of the body, at the chest and shoulder level, creep forward taking tension off the backside of the buckle *above* the apex. Over time, it results in a forward curvature in the upper half of the coils and spine. In the spring, this is comparative to the upper back, shoulders and head at the same level in the body. In the body, it is the actual hunching back, slumping shoulders and forward head posture (FHP.) It's the actual horizontal wrinkles or rolls in the low back area. It's the actual protrusion of the entire abdomen.

**Image 2.26**
**Spring with creep depicted to the area above the buckle. Body with creep depicted to the area above the buckle, or waist. Shaded profiles indicate balanced spring and body position.**

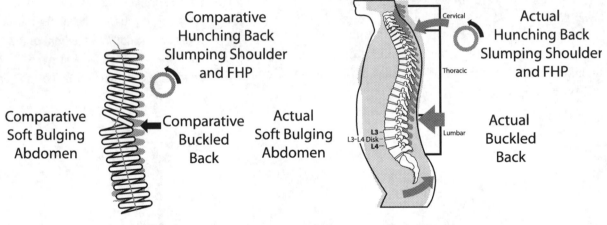

Comparative Hunching Back Slumping Shoulder and FHP

Actual Hunching Back Slumping Shoulder and FHP

Comparative Soft Bulging Abdomen

Comparative Buckled Back

Actual Soft Bulging Abdomen

Actual Buckled Back

Cervical

Thoracic

Lumbar

L3
L3-L4 Disk
L4

Above the Buckle Creep in the Spring and Body

## Creep below the buckle

Creep occurring below the buckle in the spring is comparable to creep below the L3 and L4 vertebral disk or belly button level spine in the body. The coils of the spring and vertebra of the body, at the L4, L5 and sacral level, creep forward taking tension off the backside of the buckle below the apex. In the spring, this is comparative to buttocks, tailbone and belly at the same level in the body. In the body it is the actual leaning back posture while standing or walking. In the body, it is the actual flat buttocks because the tailbone has creeped forward taking the bottom with it. They are also soft and saggy because they're hanging lifeless on locked

**Image 2.27**
**Spring with creep depicted to the area below the buckle. Body with creep depicted to the area below the buckle, or belly button level waist. The shaded profiles indicate the balanced spring and body position.**

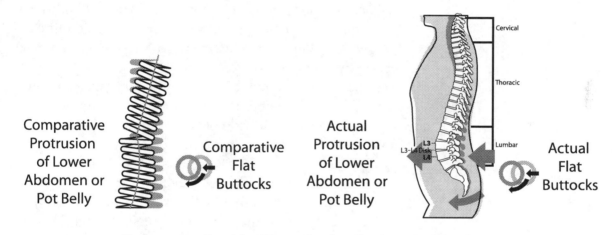

Comparative Protrusion of Lower Abdomen or Pot Belly

Comparative Flat Buttocks

Actual Protrusion of Lower Abdomen or Pot Belly

Cervical

Thoracic

Lumbar

L3
L3-L4 Disk
L4

Actual Flat Buttocks

### Below the Buckle Creep in the Spring and Body

up joints. It's the actual protrusion of the lower abdomen or potbelly. This is because the spine has creeped forward exclusively below the bellybutton-level waist. The lower abdomen moves forward with it. This is apparent even in slender people. It is the actual horizontal wrinkles or rolls in the upper abdomen just above the belly button.

## There You Have It

- The basic engineering characteristic of the spring and body;
- The basic mechanical behavior of the spring and body in response to unbalanced loads;
- Some hints on how to bury yourself in technicalities and make clear thinking impossible – if you wish.

## Some Differences between the Spring and Spine

Here are some other differences between a spring and spine.

A spring is inanimate. A body is animate. A spring can only correct misalignment by outside influence. A body heals itself through unconscious effort. It can be helped through its own conscious effort or intelligent design – sometimes called **Perfect Posture Positioning**.

The spring is not affected by whim. Only through mechanical failure does the spring alter its weight-carrying and transfer points. It will not shift its axial load because of a whimsical idea of how it should look or what is considered fashionable.

Someone may attempt to "stand up straight" or "sit up straight" in an attempt to look the way he thinks is or looks respectful, stylish, virtuous or socially appropriate. He or she may assume a posture and persona to fit a situation and find it rewarding. He or she might then maintain that posture and persona in an attempt to perpetually preserve that circumstance or role. He or she may assume a posture and then maintain that posture in an attempt to attain enlightenment. Reasons for assuming unbalanced body positions are limitless and certainly necessary at times. But, when held obsessively, or repetitively, they can alter the body's form and function.

There are also all the artifacts that are worn or used in some manner and their related aches, pains, strains and deformities. A spring does not use those either.

## Postural Debits and Credits

All this unnatural posturing is fine as long as you have the know-how to correct the alterations and develop a feel for where the body is naturally meant to be. There is a postural debit and credit sheet in everyone's body. When you stand asymmetrically, you are racking up debits on your postural account sheet. Too much time spent asymmetrically positioned and, in time, you're looking at postural bankruptcy and eventual collapse somewhere in your body. In other words muscle strain, slouching shoulders, sunken chest, hunchback or kyphosis, low back problems, saddlebags, cellulite, bad knees or hips, full protruding soft abdomen, pot belly, abdominal hernia and so on, and so on, and...you get the picture. It causes a lot of different problems.

You must spend an adequate amount of time properly positioned and vertically centered to build up postural credits. It's not a shame if you spend time standing, walking or sitting in an unbalanced manner. It is a shame if you stand, walk or sit in an unbalanced manner, and then, don't even know how to balance the body when the time comes. It's unfortunate that most people do not know where their central axis is and how to position themselves symmetrically around it. Or, they feel strongly they must stand and move in an anatomically incorrect manner at all times in order to "fit in," "look good," or even "intimidate." This book will remedy that. By showing how it's possible to maintain an anatomically correct posture, there should be no need to worry about "fitting in" or "looking good." A naturally proportioned, balanced and evenly toned posture can't help but be beautiful. When you think about it, it's the strained, tense, rigid, crooked or bulging postures that make us nervous or repel us. A posture displaying poise and quiet strength attracts us and instantly gains our respect. Desire for a naturally proportioned, balanced and evenly toned body should guide our efforts for proper posture, not whimsical notions about appearance.

You now have an understanding of how outside influences alter the body. You know the engineering characteristics of a symmetrical, balanced, evenly toned spring and body. You know the mechanical behavior of the spring and body in response to tilt.

You might say, "Yes, yes, I understand all of this bendy stuff and why it happens. It seems to make perfect sense. I saw the pictures of the spring and body with a properly positioned axis and balanced load. I understand why some buckled and creeped out." You might ask, "Exactly how does the human body assume the position that affords symmetry around the axis? Exactly how do I position my body to maintain gravity in a balanced or axial manner upon it? How do I do this so that I might be properly proportioned, balanced and evenly toned front to back and side to side from top to bottom?" Of course you might, otherwise you wouldn't have bought this book.

You'll learn the points for centering and, therefore, how to balance the body in the next chapter. Practice the progressions and imagery drills in the "how to get it and keep it" chapters. Even reading and thinking about the points of centering you'll learn is a postural credit.

# Chapter Two

# What Perfect Posture Is

## Equilibrium, Balance, Centering and Symmetry

In this chapter, you will learn how to position certain points on the body while standing or walking so you can maintain equilibrium of balance. It's the position where the pull of gravity will be evenly balanced from head to foot. It's the position where the push of the body up will be evenly balanced from foot to head. It's the position where the body is arranged around the central axis symmetrically. It then follows that stresses or tension will be equal, front to back and side to side, from top to bottom.

How to sit without damaging the spine and body is included at no extra charge.

I call these instructions "commandments" to emphasize the importance of adherence to their principles.

I call the indicated locations on the body "points of center*ing*" or "center*ing* points" because it will help you identify with the realization that posture is an action or process. You should really not even use the word *posture*. It's usually considered a noun and, therefore, the name of some*thing*. It hypnotizes you into trying to concretize a look, a pose or fixed position. Instead of saying someone has good *posture*, you really should be saying, someone has good postur*ing*, thereby making it a verb or action word. This would help you realize that posture is an activity or process. I will refer to posture and other associated words as verbs frequently. It will help you to identify with the concept that an action is, or should be, taking place.

Whenever I hear someone talk about a perfect or correct way of doing anything, including how to stand, I'm always a bit skeptical. So I'm a little embarrassed when I insist on strict rules of where these points on the body should be positioned. But, just a little. All bodies are basically built and behave the same so there's little freedom to move much outside these guidelines and still maintain a good posture.

There will always be disagreement over some fine tuning of the points of centering. For instance, some might say the feet should be at a 35 and not 30 degree angle from each other. Some might feel the front view line for the point of centering on the foot should run through the big toe, not the second toe.

I think these commandments for centering the body are the ideal. I tried to put them in order of importance. The first one: keeping your knees unlocked is **absolutely essential**. There is no way you can reach the reward of Perfect Posture with habitually locked knees and buckled spine. The other commandments: shoulders relaxed; ears, shoulders, hips and ankles aligned in the side view; outside of hips and knees directly vertical to the second toe in the front view. These are merely **essential**. Approximate as best you can with minor variation if you feel it's right. But if you stay reasonably close to these guidelines and keep your knees unlocked, you just about can't go wrong.

Here's something to remember. At times you will revert back to your old way of standing. You always will. You will never, repeat, *never* be able to adhere to these commandments completely, always, and in every respect. Don't try *too* hard. You'll go crazy.

Crazy does not display poise and quiet strength.
You may want to look especially cute, virtuous, respectful, upstanding or even intimidating, so you "strike a pose." Or, you may just forget and find you're standing in the old way. This is fine. But when the moment passes, get back into the balanced position you're going to learn. In time, it won't feel odd or uncomfortable. You'll do it unconsciously most of the time, like any habit you pick up. Your legs won't get tired so fast. You'll feel as normal balancing your upper body on your legs with your knees unlocked as you did with your old way of standing. You'll feel poised and relaxed. You'll look so good and will hear about it so much it will always be on

your mind. You won't feel the need to contort and *hold* your body in a rigid position because you'll know you're looking the best that you can when you're centered.

Get the following commandments memorized. Incorporate the "how to get it" and "how to keep it" chapters into your daily activities. In time, your kinesthesia - the perception or sensing of the motion, weight and position of the body as muscles, tendons, and joints move in these positions - will be familiar and comfortable. In time, you'll have the body you knew you were meant to have.

Don't get too excited. Relax those shoulders.

Below are the ten commandments of Perfect Posture body mechanics for standing as laid down by Mother Nature. An explanation of each will follow. Learn them and live by them or suffer the wrath of… Mother Nature.

Or don't. You'll have a less than perfect body. That's all. Don't worry. Don't fret. You won't go to that bad place when you die. (The only way that will happen is if somehow you're reading this book without paying for it.)

But, as long as you've got to live your life, why not be the best that you can be with the minimal amount of effort? The simple effort of habit. The best you can be without obsessive, compulsive, sweaty, inconvenient exercise that doesn't work that well anyway.

---

# Commandments for Standing

1. **Never lock your knees**
2. **Shoulders relaxed at all times**
3. **Earlobes vertical to the middle of your shoulders in the side view**
4. **Middle of shoulder vertical to the hipbone in the side view**
5. **Hipbone vertical to the anklebone in the side view**
6. **Earlobe, mid-shoulder, hipbone, and anklebone vertically aligned in the side view**
7. **Outside of the hips vertical to the outside of the knees in the frontal view**
8. **Outside of the knee vertical to the second toe in the frontal view**
9. **Outside of hip, outside of knee, second toe vertically aligned in the frontal view**
10. **Feet at a 30-degree angle from each other**

---

## 1. Never lock your knees

There are no known facts explaining why people lock their knees back and stand too straight. What we do know for a fact is that when they do, it immediately does three things:

A) It buckles the lumbar spine to the front.

B) It stretches the abdominal wall in the same shape as the spine. Muscles habitually kept in a stretched position become weakened.

C) It tips the pelvis forward. The pelvis can be thought of as a bowl, which, if tipped, spills its contents over the edge.

Thus, with the knees locked back, the spine will push and the pelvis will spill the innards forward against a weakened belly wall. The harder the knees are locked up and the more firmly the body is held in the "up straight" position, the more forward is the push from the buckled back. The bigger is the spill from the tipped pelvis against the increasingly weakened belly wall. [Image 3.02] The way most people stand, no wonder it's almost impossible to have a flat stomach.

The problems with the back, pelvis and abdomen are just the start. The habit of locking the knees back and resting the weight of the upper body on the knees, hip joints and low back is the most damaging and the most common of the habits that make for a deformed or "old" body. [Image 3.02] All the weight of the upper body is supported by the knee joint, the hip joint, the low back and various ligaments. As odd as it sounds, your legs and buttocks muscles are not holding you up at all. They're just limply hanging on the locked up hip and knee joints, almost like they're paralyzed. *Some* of the other problems stemming from locked knees are flat flabby buttocks, saddlebags, cellulite and shapeless ankles.

If you unlock your knees, your back will assume its natural, less exaggerated arch and your pelvis will resume its balanced, level position. [Image 3.03] How quickly depends on the time spent out of center and how far. The spine will no longer be pushing, and the pelvis spilling, the intestines

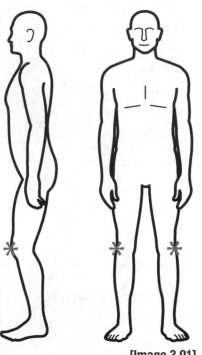

**[Image 3.01]**
**Unlock the knees.**

forward. The innards will no longer push and spill against a chronically stretched and weakened belly wall. Time-dependent creep will no longer be creeping. The difficult part will be having the patience and fortitude to keep the knees unlocked while your legs are getting stronger. Shift weight from foot to foot, lean on something, dance the box step, sit down, get up, shift weight forward and back. Your body is not built to stand stationary anyway. Don't try to cheat nature by locking your knees. Nature will win. Your abdomen will be soft and protrude. You will have, or get, those other unwanted features and probably more.

The only remedy is monotonous, painful exercise to strengthen and shorten the stomach muscles. And even with exercise, diet or both, you will still have that annoying little potbelly. When no longer inspired by some fitness cheerleader or other, the belly will come back like before. Wouldn't it make more sense to just take the time during your everyday activities to get in the habit of standing correctly? You would be eliminating the problems once and for all.

Unlock those knees and keep them unlocked. Don't go to extremes except when practicing in private. You don't need to drag your knuckles on the ground or walk like Groucho Marx. People that know you well or see you on a daily basis may notice at first. But, they'll get used to it. You'll get used to it. The comments will cease. Barely unlocked does the trick. The knees will only be moving 2-3 inches from where they used to be. Get the buckle out of your back and your pelvis level. Put the contents of your stomach where they belong, resting in the leveled pelvic bowl, not pushed and spilled out the front. It may take some time, depending on your overall condition. Your legs may get tired or quivery but that doesn't mean you should lock your knees to rest on locked-up joints. It means you should lean on a wall with your knees unlocked and the small of your back pressed against it. It means you should pace or waltz in a little circle, practicing the walking commandments you'll learn. Keep a folding stool handy. Sit down for a moment, then start all over. If possible, sit on the ground. In the long run, your

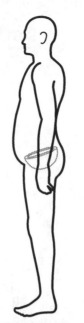

[Image 3.02]
**The pelvis tips forward like a bowl.**

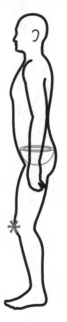

[Image 3.03]
**The pelvis is level with unlocked knees.**

body will thank you for it with an unbuckled low back, flat abdomen and all the rest that goes with it.

All the remaining commandments will be explained with the taking for granted that you are standing with your knees unlocked.

## 2. Shoulders relaxed at all times

If you lock your knees back and "stand up straight," with your "chest out, stomach in, and chin up", you're *holding* your shoulders in an unbalanced fashion. The human body, therefore the spine, is a composite of balanced forces. When you attempt to *hold* yourself in a certain manner, stresses become unbalanced. You interrupt the natural, balanced flow of tonus coursing through the body. As holding becomes habitual, it will begin to feel normal. Your body knows where it is meant to be. If you have your knees unlocked and the points of centering accurately position**ing**, it will go there if given the chance. Any attempt to "hold" the body in a fixed manner will alter the pitch of the vertebrae and the space between them. The spine will become habituated and feel normal or natural in a large deformation. It is not normal, or natural. As with the spring, the spine will experience the inevitable time-dependent creep and will begin to bend in order to distribute the stresses more evenly over the cross sections of the vertebrae. No matter what your diet, exercise, determination or virtuous intent, Mother Nature and gravity will win. The spine will become abnormally or unnaturally bent and crooked. Let the shoulders relax. Let the upper body relax on top of the pelvis, the pelvis resting on the unlocked legs. [Image 3.04] The spine will become, or stay, properly pitched and angled, the body along with it will become, or stay, naturally balanced, arched and evenly toned.

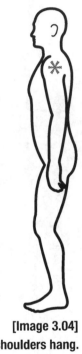

**[Image 3.04]**
**Just let the shoulders hang.**

### 3. Earlobes vertical to the middle of your shoulders in the side view

Keeping your head centered over your shoulders is not something you would think anyone would need to be told about. But if you look around and listen, it's obvious this isn't so. With the many examples of people with heads held too far forward and complaints of sore necks, it's best included in this book. Since people don't have eyes in the sides of their heads, it's difficult to see if you are habitually noncompliant with this commandment. A friend would have to look or take a picture from the side. Better yet, just practice the centering exercises in the "how to get it" chapter and develop a feeling for correctness. If you keep yourself aware of your other centering points, and center the head frequently, it will eventually migrate back to the centered position. The earlobe will be even with the midline of the shoulders. [Image 3.05] Then, if you keep your legs unlocked and occasionally center your head and body, it will stay there.

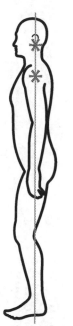

**[Image 3.05]**
**Earlobes vertical to shoulder.**

### 4. Middle of the shoulder vertical to the hipbone in the side view

A vertical straight line should run from the hipbone to the middle of the shoulder. [Image 3.06]

If you're used to standing too straight with the knees locked back, despite your best intentions, your shoulders are probably routinely forward or back of this line. Your back is likely hunching forward or leaning to the back of this line. It will feel awkward at first to unlock your knees and let your back and shoulders relax. But, think of the time spent out of center and the solidity of the tissues that have to change. It took some time to get the way you are. Take some time to get used to it and correct those stiff and rigid tissues.

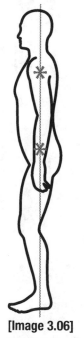

**[Image 3.06]**
**Shoulder vertical to hip.**

## 5. Hipbone vertical to the anklebone in the side view

You see a lot of hips outside the vertical center of gravity. It shows how the individual consciously, or the body unconsciously, adjusts to increased stresses in the rear side of the lower spine.

With shoulders relaxed and knees slightly bent, the hips should be positioned directly above the anklebone. [Image 3.07] This may feel very awkward or funny at first if your habits have been poor and your spine is out of its natural shape.

## 6. Earlobe, mid-shoulder, hipbone, and anklebone vertically aligned in the side view

Number six is basically a summary of #3, #4 and #5. A straight line should run *directly* vertical from the ankle through the hip to the mid shoulder, through the earlobe and out the top of the head. [Image 3.08] Keep the shoulders relaxed. It may feel odd depending on time and habits. (Yes, you're probably sick of hearing how funny it's going to feel standing correctly, but you must be prepared for this). The more off center, and time spent that way, the odder it will feel. Remember you probably got used to standing incorrectly at a very young age. Your back is probably stiff and deformed. It will take a substantial amount of time to feel normal standing correctly. It will take time for your back to migrate or correct to the straighter, balanced position. You can speed the process by doing the limbering progressions in the "how to get it" chapter. But remember, you are dealing with bone, ligaments and cartilage. These tissues do not change overnight. Take it slow. Be patient!

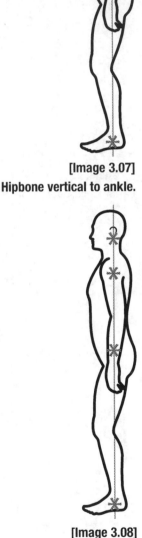

**[Image 3.07]**
**Hipbone vertical to ankle.**

**[Image 3.08]**
**Earlobe vertical to shoulder,**
**hip and ankle.**

### 7. Outside of the hips vertical to the outside of the knees in the frontal view

A vertical line should run from the outside of the hip to the outside of the knee for reasons that are explained, in depth, following commandment number nine. [Image 3.09]

### 8. Outside of the knee vertical to the second toe in the frontal view

A vertical line should run from the outside of the knee through the second toe for reasons that are explained, in depth, following commandment number nine. [Image 3.10]

### 9. Outside of hip, outside of knee, second toe, vertically aligned in the frontal view

#9 is basically a summary of #7 and #8.
It stands to reason that if your feet are the width of your hips, your knees will be too. Not always so, but usually. If repetition helps you learn, then this redundancy will serve its purpose. It's essential you know where these sites are, so there is no question about where your points of centering are located. A straight, *directly* vertical line should run from the second toe to the outside of the knee to the outside of the hip. It shouldn't angle left or angle right.

The reasons why it is so important to have the feet correctly positioned are explained below. [Image 3.11]

### Why the feet need to be accurately positioned

When you habitually stand with your feet too close together or too far apart, you further contribute to the existing problems caused by locking the knees. These include, but are not limited to, flabby buttocks, cellulite and especially so-called saddlebags and love handles. It also increases the risk of injury to the sacroiliac joint, causing sciatica, which is characterized by pain and tenderness in the very low back

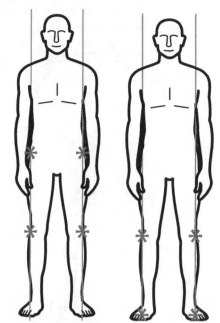

[Image 3.09 & 3.10]
**Outside of hips vertical to outside of knees. Outside of knee vertical to second toe.**

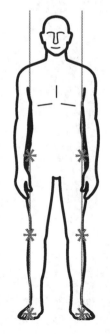

[Image 3.11]
**Outside of hip vertical to outside of knee and second toe.**

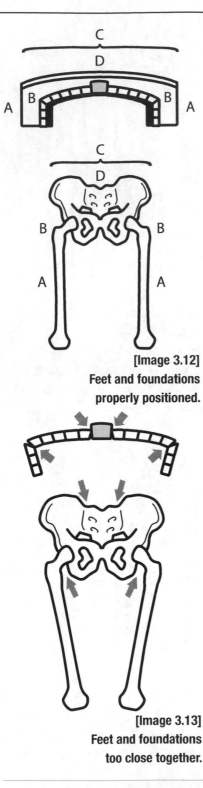

[Image 3.12]
Feet and foundations
properly positioned.

[Image 3.13]
Feet and foundations
too close together.

or upper buttocks. The pain can also radiate down the legs. If you have sciatica, you probably have a long history of holding the feet at an incorrect angle and too close together or far apart.

To make the reasons for this understandable, I'll again model a biological form after a non-biological structure that's built and behaves comparably. This example will use a stone bridge for the model.

In this comparison, the feet will relate to the foundations of the bridge (not shown). The legs will be compared to the supports (A). The hips will represent the cornerstones (B). The pelvis will be compared to the arch of the bridge (C), and the sacroiliac to the keystone of the bridge (D). [Image 3.12]

When you stand with your feet too close together or too far apart you weaken the physical structure of the body. It's weakened in the same way a bridge would be if its foundations were moved too far in or out. The further and longer the foundations are out of position, the worse the damage. The worse the damage, the harder to fix, be it bridge or body.

For a bridge to move its foundations in or out would require some sort of adverse occurrence, say an earthquake or flood, for instance. Like the spring, the bridge won't surrender its structural integrity because of a whimsical idea of how it should look.

### Supports and feet too close together

If the support foundations of the bridge are somehow moved too close together, the supports are angled *out* from the bottom. It causes the arch to *sag* and *widen*. This puts extra pressure on the upper part of the keystone and the lower parts of the cornerstones. [Image 3.13] It will destabilize the structural integrity of the keystone, arch and cornerstones. It can eventually cause the keystone and cornerstones to crumble and the bridge to collapse.

It's the same with the pelvis and the legs. If the feet are habitually held too close together, the legs are angled *out* from the bottom. It causes the pelvic arch to *sag* and *widen*. This puts extra pressure on the upper part of the sacroiliac and the lower part of the hip joints. It will destabilize the structural integrity of the sacroiliac, pelvis and hips. It can eventually cause inflammation of the sacroiliac and hips, and debilitating pain. In the meantime, it contributes to flabby buttocks and hips with the pronounced saddlebags originating at the bottom of the hip joint. The structural issues are not restricted to the sacroiliac, pelvis and hips. The unbalanced forces result in offset or uneven compression effects on the knees and ankles also. If habitual, it can cause inflammation and eventually breakdown of these joints as well.

### Supports and feet too far apart

If the support foundations of the bridge are moved too far apart, the supports are angled *in* from the bottom. It causes the arch to increase its arc *upward* and to *narrow*. This puts extra pressure on the lower part of the keystone and the upper parts of the cornerstones. It will destabilize the structural integrity of the keystone, arch and cornerstones. [Image 3.14] It also can eventually cause the keystone and cornerstones to crumble and the bridge to collapse.

Again, it's the same with the pelvis and legs. If the feet are habitually held too far apart, the legs are angled *in* from the bottom. It causes the pelvic arch to increase its arc *upward* and to *narrow*. This puts extra pressure on the lower part of the sacroiliac and the upper part of the hip joints. It will destabilize the structural integrity of the sacroiliac, pelvis and hips. It can eventually cause inflammation of the sacroiliac and hips, and debilitating pain. In the meantime, it contributes to flabby buttocks and hips with the pronounced saddlebags originating at the top of the hip joint. The structural issues are not restricted to the sacroiliac, pelvis and hips. The unbalanced forces result in offset or uneven compression effects on the knees and ankles also. If habitual, it can cause inflammation and eventually breakdown of these joints as well.

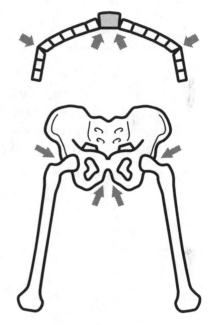

[Image 3.14]
**Feet and foundations too far apart.**

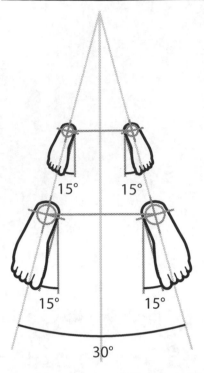

**[Image 3.15]**
Habitually standing with too much or too little angle will result in chronic torsion stress on the hips and knees.

### 10. Feet at a 30-degree angle from each other

This position for the feet is for stability. Too little angle between them and you're unstable side to side. Too much angle and you're unstable front to back. Incorrect angle also causes torsion stresses on the hips, knees and ankles. The line of reference should run from the middle of the heel through the second toe. [Image 3.15]

## Commandments for Walking

It's not going to do you a lot of good to know how to stand, without hurting your body, if you don't know how to walk, without hurting your body. Therefore, I present the commandments for a walking Perfect Posture. Below you see the commandments of walking body mechanics as laid down by Mother Nature.

---

### Commandments Of Walking Body Mechanics

1. **Do not snap the knee to the locked position with the forward stride**
2. **Shoulders relaxed at all times**
3. **Don't drop, plop, or thud from leg to leg on weight transfer**
4. **Opposite shoulder vertical to anklebone at weight transfer**

---

### 1. Do not snap the knee to the locked position with the forward stride.

It buckles the spine and compresses it even more with weight transfer.

### 2. Shoulders relaxed at all times.

If not relaxed and centered, you again have the weight being transferred to an uncentered spine. This will further promote buckle and creep.

## 3. Don't drop, plop or thud from leg to leg on weight transfer

If the weight transfer is not smooth, you are locking your knees and buckling your back at the completion of your forward stride. You are *dropping* all of your weight onto the weight-bearing heel, hipbone, back and surrounding structure. It's coming down from the distance you lifted it in the apex of your stride. That's the distance, or height, from the ball of your foot to your heel at weight transfer. It's bad, bad and bad for the body. Not only is your hip joint and surrounding structure carrying all the weight of your upper body, you have the added trauma of the body falling upon them. The weight transfer should be smooth with no bouncing or jarring. When your heel comes down on the floor in your forward stride, it should not make a lot of noise or rattle the house. [Image 3.16]

## 4. Opposite shoulder vertical to anklebone at weight transfer

To keep your axis central and not throw your axial load out of balance, you need to maintain your opposite shoulders evenly above the opposite anklebones. This means, when your left foot is in the forward position of your stride, your right shoulder should be even with it from the side view. Your right shoulder should be even with your left anklebone in the rear and vice versa, with a smooth non-bouncing, non-jarring transfer of weight. [Image 3.16] This is an ideal you can only achieve when practicing. Expect perfect form only when practicing with small steps.

**[Image 3.16]**
Note how the opposite ankle is not vertical to the shoulder on the rear foot. Form will become imperfect with accelerated, longer strides and unconscious movement. Worry about perfection only when practicing. See page 104 "Doing the Crouch" image 6.10 on how to position oneself just prior to, and during walking.

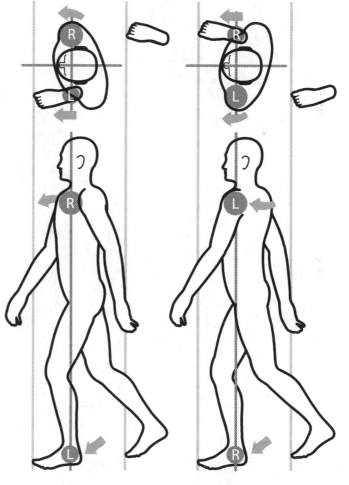

## Commandment for Sitting

Sitting and *holding* oneself *up straight* in a straight backed chair is as damaging to the back as standing and *holding* oneself *up straight* with the knees locked back. It's as damaging for the exact same reasons. It causes the low back to buckle and the pelvis to tip forward as described in Chapter One. It's more time-dependent creep in progress. [Image 3.17] There's only one commandment for sitting.

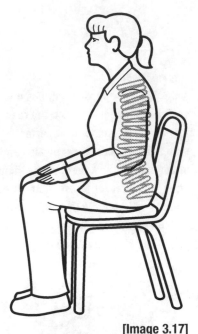

**[Image 3.17]**
**In a straight back chair the spine initially buckles and in time creep progresses. The spine develops an unbalanced pitch and angle, as illustrated by the spring overlay.**

---

### Commandment For Sitting

1. **Never sit in a chair that is reclined at less than 120 degrees**

---

This commandment is nearly impossible to keep if you're going to ride in a car, take almost any form of public transportation, work at any sit-down job or sit in any public place in the western world. It's a good example of a commandment you just cannot always keep. All you can really do is tolerate racking up postural debits and recline, recline, recline when you get the chance. Feign a bad back and slouch if you can. If you've been standing for a long time and you feel you must sit down to rest in a straight back chair, do so. You can rest your legs for a time, get back up and fidget. If circumstance allows, you can sit on the floor or ground.

When you sit on the floor or ground as illustrated, the pitch, angle and spaces of the vertebrae are at the balanced position. [Image 3.18] This is the position where tensions are equally balanced for the length of the spine - front to back, side to side, from top to bottom. The pelvic bowl is level and there is no buckle to the spine. Since there is no buckle, there will be no creep. If you lean to the front, the pelvis stays level and the low back is stretched or unbuckled forward. If you lean backwards or to the sides, the load is supported by the arms and the stress on the spine is greatly reduced. It's difficult to do much damage to the spine

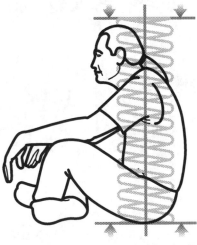

**[Image 3.18]**
**A balanced spring and a balanced spine do not tilt, buckle or creep.**

when sitting on the floor or ground. Remember, this can be uncomfortable, even painful if your low back is used to being buckled, as the disks are compressed on the backside of the spine. Taking the pressure off too fast can hurt. It doesn't mean you're doing the wrong thing. It means you're doing the *right thing too fast* and not giving your back time to adjust. These are bones, ligaments and cartilage. They don't change or heal overnight. Be patient in the idea that you are doing the right thing, but do it slowly. Don't discourage yourself. Get use to a stretched out back slowly. Practice the progressions you'll learn in Chapter Four when you can.

## Fidgeting Leg to Leg

If you are going to stand for extended periods, you're going to need to shift weight from leg to leg to rest. If you are going to shift weight leg to leg, you need to know how to do it and keep your axis positioned and load balanced.

Sorry, you can't.

But, since you will be doing this, as everyone does and needs to, it would be good to have some guidelines so you do as little damage as possible. Therefore, the comandments for fidgeting [Image 3.19]:

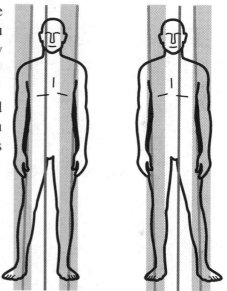

---

### Commandments For Fidgeting Leg To Leg

1. **Never lock your knee back on the weight bearing leg**
2. **Never let one of the side view centering points be more than 3 inches out of center**
3. **Never let one of the front view centering points be more than 3 inches out of center**

---

[Image 3.19]
When supporting on one leg, remember to keep your points of center within three inches of the centered zone – front to back and side to side.

That's it. If you stay reasonably close to these guidelines, you'll do little damage habitually standing on one leg at a time. If you only go three inches out of centering front to back or side to side, that's three inches on each side of center. Added together, that's six inches of wobble room.

It should be enough for an incredibly striking pose. Just make sure you don't get in the habit of standing on one side only always, or you'll develop the problem of scoliosis (same cause and effect, just sideways.) Shift leg to leg often and try to keep the amount of time spent on each one equal.

## Concentration

The simple effort of concentrating on standing, moving and sitting correctly until it becomes an unconscious habit is all it takes. Take the time to get used to standing, moving and sitting in a non-harmful manner. Your body will stay properly proportioned and evenly toned front to back and side to side, from top to bottom just by force of habit. It will be no more difficult or tiring than your current way of standing, moving or sitting.

Your legs were built for this. You get tired now when you stand too long. You'll get tired with your new way of standing also. You just won't be damaging your body in the process. Eventually, like any habit, you'll do it without thinking. Once you've gotten your back unbuckled, the pelvis leveled and the leg muscles strong enough to hold you up for prolonged periods, Perfect Posturing will be automatic. You'll do it without thinking, except for occasional maintenance. The change-over may take some time. It's relative to how old you are and how unbalanced your habits have been. You'll get better and better at knowing, inside your head, when you are positioning in balance with the laws of Mother Nature. Keeping these commandments holy or, even partially, will help you lose many undesirable characteristics. The next chapter will explain some of the characteristics you can lose practicing the commandments of Perfect Posturing.

Start your children on these principles at an early age so they won't have to go through the process of adjustment.

# Chapter Three
# What Perfect Posture Can Do

## Taking Some Close-ups

In this chapter, particular characteristics and body parts will be examined. What can be done with these characteristics and parts when you maintain a habit of centered posturing will be explained. In the movie business, this would be called taking some close-ups.

I'll start at the top and work my way down.

**Height increase**

If you tilt the load on a spring off its axis, you buckle the spring. The spring is shortened by this occurrence. [Image 4.01]  If the weight shift is prolonged, repetitive or both, you also get time-dependent creep. This further shortens the spring. [Image 4.02] It's the same with a body. If you tilt the load on a body off its axis by locking the knees, you buckle the spine. The spine and, therefore, the body are shortened. If the weight shift is prolonged, repetitive or both, you also get creep. This further shortens the spine and body. It shortens in the identical way, according to the same mechanical behavior and effects of nature as the spring.

If you correct the unbalanced load on a spring, it would rebound to an extent relative to how far and how long it had been out of balance, buckled and creeped. Permanent set may have occurred and it will never resume its original shape and height.

If you correct the unbalanced load on a spine, it has a much greater ability to rebound to the position it would have been if it had never been out of balance, buckled and creeped.  Unlike the spring, the spine can heal or correct itself to pre-buckle, pre-creep and pre-shortened conditions.

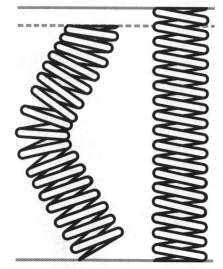

[Image 4.01]
**Unbalance load buckles spring, shortens height.**

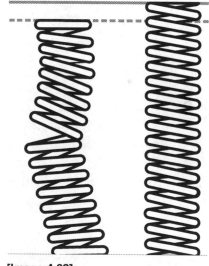

[Image 4.02]
**With time creep occurs and further shortens height.**

When you stand with your knees unlocked, your spine will lose the buckle at the lower back and gain some height. If you've been standing locked up for a considerable amount of time, you must also lose the time-dependent creep. It will take a considerable amount of time. How fast depends on the duration and intensity of the previous unbalanced habits, and the duration and intensity of effort you put into quitting those habits. Correcting the creep will further straighten the spine, further increasing height. Depending on many factors, you can expect to gain between one and three inches in height with Perfect Posture. [Image 4.03]

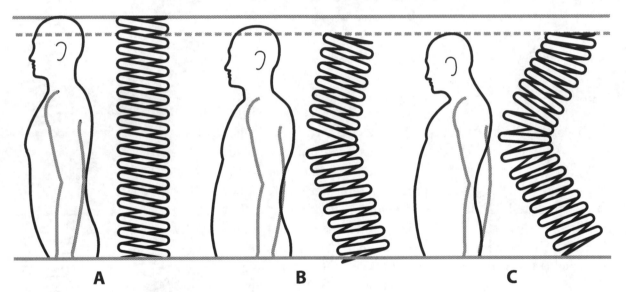

**A**        **B**        **C**

[Image 4.03]
(A) The balanced spring and body at full height.
(B) The buckled, shortened spring and body.
(C) The buckled, creeped and further shortened spring and body.

## Forward head posture

The head creeping forward is a continuation of the overly forward curved upper back. With the knees unlocked, the waist-level spine will unbuckle and tone will become, or start to become, equal front and back. The process of buckle and creep will reverse. The upper back will respond and become straighter as stresses are equalized on both sides of the spine. With the shoulders relaxed directly above the hips and ankles, gravity will become, or start to become, balanced. The head will then migrate back to its proper position along with the upper back. It will be centered with the earlobe vertical to the straightened shoulders. [Image 4.04]

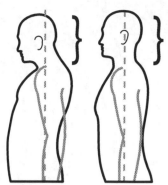

[Image 4.04]
**Forward head creep and Perfect Posture comparison.**

## Forward-curved upper back or above-waist creep

This is also known as kyphosis, or dowager's hump. This is the primary characteristic of above-the-waist creep. It is associated with a visibly high degree of forward arch to the low back. With the knees unlocked and points centered, the low back will lose, or start to lose, its buckle. As stresses become, or start to become, equal front and back of the waist-level spine, the upper back will respond. The process of buckle and creep as described in Chapter One will reverse itself. Stresses become, or start to become, equal front and back of the upper spine. The upper back will loose, or start to loose, its forward curve, becoming straighter as stresses are equalized the entire length of the spine. [Image 4.05]

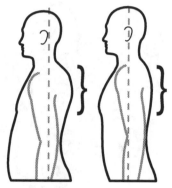

[Image 4.05]
**Slouched shoulders and Perfect Posture comparison.**

## Slumping shoulders

Over time, the upper spine creeps forward for the reasons stated in Chapter One. The back follows the spine and the shoulders follow the back. With the knees unlocked and the points centered, the process of buckle and creep will reverse. The shoulders will migrate to the rear along with the upper back and spine. [Image 4.06]

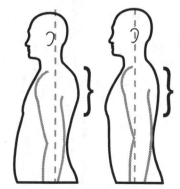

[Image 4.06]
**Slumping Shoulders in comparison with Perfect Posture.**

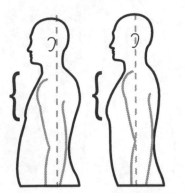

**[Image 4.07]**
**Sunken chest in comparison with Perfect Posture.**

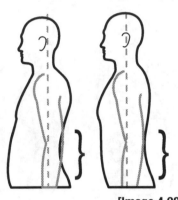

**[Image 4.08]**
**Swayback in comparison with Perfect Posture.**

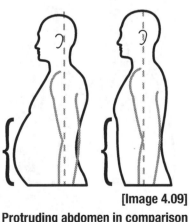

**[Image 4.09]**
**Protruding abdomen in comparison with Perfect Posture.**

## Sunken chest

The chest, like the shoulders, abdomen or any part of the body's trunk, follows the lead of the spine. After the low back buckles, the upper spine creeps forward. The chest follows the shape of the upper spine. It sinks into a concave shape. With the knees unlocked and the points centered, the process of buckle and creep reverse. The spine will become, or start to become, straightened. The chest follows the straightened upper spine and assumes a more convex or outward arched shape. The shoulders are positioned well behind the chest in the side view with Perfect Posture. [Image 4.07]

## Buckled, overarched, swayback, lordotic low back

The low back is the point where the troubles with posture begin when you lock the knees. By now, you're well aware of the fact that locking the knees causes a buckling of the waist-level back. The further, harder and longer the knees are locked back, the more the buckle. If you unlocked the knees, the low back would unbuckle, or start to. You would lose some arch to the low back. You would lose or start to lose all the physical alterations associated with this habit. [Image 4.08]

## Full length protruding abdomen

The abdomen, like the shoulders, chest or any part of the trunk, follows the lead of the spine. Full length protruding abdomen is characteristic of *above*-the-waist creep. The reason the *entire* abdomen protrudes is because the *entire* abdominal area, top to bottom, is evenly pushed to the front in a big long curve by *all* of the lumbar vertebrae (see Chapter 4, Part 1). With the knees unlocked and points centered, the spine will unbuckle and the intestines will follow. The pelvic bowl will tilt back in the leveled position, with the intestines no longer spilling out the front. The abdomen flattens out and has normal tonus flowing through it rather than bulging out and being soft. The abdomen is flat and proportioned in the side view of the Perfect Posture illustration. [Image 4.09]

## Under-arched, flat low back or hypolordosis

The low back is the point where the troubles with posture begin when you lock the knees. You should be aware (sick and tired?) of the fact that locking the knees causes a buckling of the waist-level back. A waist-level back, with an apparently low or *flat* degree of arch, is characteristic of below-the-waist creep. This is because the back below the L3- 4 disk has only 2 disks, or joints, and 3 bones to creep or *curl* forward relieving pressure on the posterior spine. These three joints move forward almost like a single unit, without much of a curve. It's hard to see. It just makes the low back *look* flat.

If you unlocked your knees, tension in the lumbar spine would become, or start to become, equal front to back. It would become unbuckled. The spine below the L 3- 4 disk would respond, equalizing tension. It would reverse the forward creep as described in Chapter 1 and move posterior. You would develop a balanced, proper, more *visible* arch to the low back. You would get some tone and roundness to the buttocks. You would develop a balanced posture and wouldn't seem to be leaning back all the time. [Image 4.10]

## Partially protruding abdomen (potbelly)

The abdomen, like the shoulders, chest or any part of the trunk, follows the lead of the spine. Partially protruding abdomen (potbelly) is characteristic of *below* the waist creep. This is because the spine, *below* the L3- 4 spinal disks or belly button level waist, has creeped anteriorly. This gives the abdominal area *below* the belly button an extra push out the front. Hence, you have the "pot" out forward of the rest of the abdominal area above the belly button. Unlock the knees, unbuckle the back, loose the below the buckle creep. Problem solved. [Image 4.11]

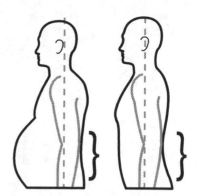
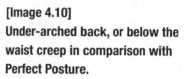

[Image 4.10]
**Under-arched back, or below the waist creep in comparison with Perfect Posture.**

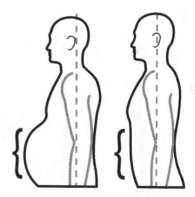

[Image 4.11]
**Partially protruding abdomen (potbelly).**

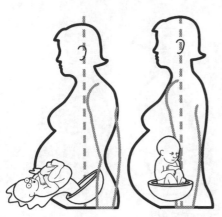

**[Image 4.12]**
**Pregnancy, protruding abdomen and posture.**

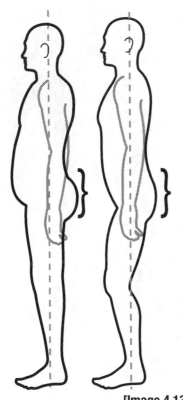

**[Image 4.13]**
**Flabby, soft and/or round bottom with above the waist creep in comparison with Perfect Posture.**

## Pregnancy, protruding abdomen and posture

As long as I'm on the subject of protruding abdomen, it would be a good time to address the issue of pregnancy. If you are a woman who locks your knees back and is pregnant, or thinking about becoming so, consider all of the dynamics explained. Now, consider adding, at a minimum, 30 pounds to the contents of your pelvic bowl. If you do not, or cannot, practice Perfect Posture you have, or will have, all of that extra weight pushing and spilling up against your abdominal wall. It is, or will be, pushing and spilling against an abdominal wall that is triple stretched and weakened. It will be stretched and weakened from the buckled spine, the tipped pelvis *and* the volume of a baby as well. Bad, bad, and triple bad for the abdominal wall. Try to get used to standing centered with the knees unlocked before you get pregnant. If already pregnant, stand centered with the knees unlocked as much as you possibly can. Then, recline, recline, recline in a properly angled chair when you can't.

I won't bring up what all that extra unbalanced weight can do to a buckled spine and the rest of your body. Think about it. [Image 4.12]

## Soft or toneless *round* bottom

Another side effect of locking the knees and resting the weight of the upper body on the low back, hip and knee joints is the relaxation of the buttocks and leg muscles. This will cause flabby or soft buttocks. Round buttocks are characteristic of above-the-waist creep. They're round because the spine below the waist stays buckled all the way back – no forward creep. The reason they're flabby is because they are not doing the work of holding you up. They're hanging limp on locked-up joints. With centered posturing, this can be a problem of the past. You can feel the result immediately if you unlock your knees, relax your shoulders and assume a centered position. Make sure your feet are hip width and at a 30-degree angle. Pinch or squeeze your bottom while you do this. You'll be able to feel the tone return to your buttocks. Flab and softness will be gone. They will stay gone if you take the time to learn the commandments, practice them, and make it a habit. [Image 4.13]

## Soft or toneless *flat* bottom

The buttocks, like the shoulders, abdomen or any part of the body's trunk, follows the lead of the spine. Flabby and flat buttocks are especially notable if creep is predominantly *below* the waist.

The reason they appear flat is because they have creeped forward with the spine below the L3- 4 vertebral disk. With the knees unlocked and points centered, the buttocks will migrate back to the posterior with the spine, becoming rounder and toned. You can feel the result immediately if you do the pinch or squeeze drill from the preceding close-up.

Assuming Perfect Posture positioning would create a rounder, more contoured bottom. This will also cause an increase in height, straightened shoulders, forward positioned chest and a more neutral, upright stature. [Image 4.14]

## Cankles

This is a condition in which the calves seem to extend all the way to the feet. It's a sort of combination of calves and ankles. Hence, the term: Cankles. The reason they occur is the same as for the rest of the lower-extremity muscles: Non use. With the knees locked, the ankles are flaccid, like the buttocks, hips and thighs. The ankles are not doing much of anything as far as balance and stress equalization goes. They basically exist at the bottom of your legs, atrophying or degenerating and filling with fluid. Cankles are most common in people with above-the-waist creep and **solidly** locked back knees. They usually have an especially high arch to the low back, prominent or rounded **soft** buttocks, cellulite and rounded shoulders as they age.

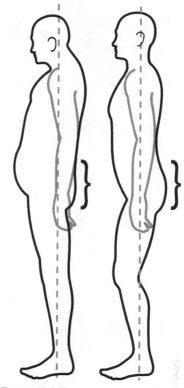

**[Image 4.14]**
**Flabby, soft and/or flat bottom with below the waist creep in comparison with Perfect Posture.**

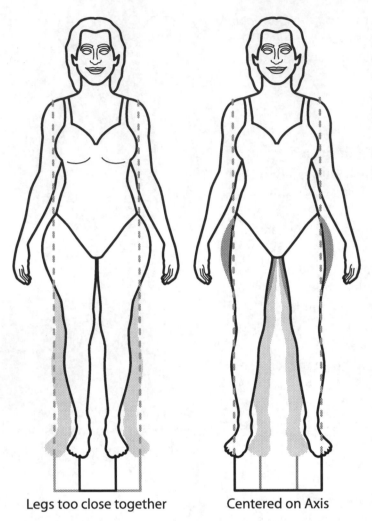

Legs too close together | Centered on Axis

**[Image 4.15]**
**Saddlebags are the gathering of shortened, limp muscles and fat around the hip area due to locked knees. They are enhanced by legs positioned off the frontal points of centering.**

Unlock those knees, position those points and make it a habit. Those cankles will get some shape, helping the legs hold you up and keeping stresses balanced. You'll find you have ankles after all.

### Saddlebags or flabby bulges on the hip

Saddlebags are another side effect of locking the knees. It's most notable in women. In the example, the feet are also too close together, further contributing to the problem as explained in commandment #9. Do the same drill as with the flabby buttocks. Pinch or squeeze your hips or saddlebags, unlock the knees, assume the commandment positioning. Feel that resting tonus in your hips where the saddlebags used to be. That is the tone and shape your upper thighs and hips were created to have. Accustom yourself to a centered posturing. Your legs will get strong. They will get used to it. It will become as effortless as your current way of standing. You won't have saddlebags. You'll be a babe. You'll have to get used to that too. [Image 4.15] Keep the feet at the proper width and angle.

### Cellulite

Locked knees are the main, if not the only, cause of cellulite. The degree this condition affects you is proportionate to how tightly the knees are locked back and the amount of time spent that way. It doesn't matter if you are tall, short, narrow or wide. Cellulite is a condition resulting from flaccid muscle tissue in your legs and buttocks. You are very much used to being held upright by tightly locked-up joints and ligaments. Your legs and buttocks muscles are not really doing much of anything, except limply hanging on the bones and soaking up fluids like a sponge.

If you are highly affected by cellulite, you'll have an especially hard time learning to habitually stand with the knees unlocked because your legs are so weak. It will feel especially odd standing in a balanced manner because your senses are especially unfamiliar with these positions. It will take especially long to get your legs strong enough to hold you for extended periods. Start out slow. Unlock the knees and stand centered for five minutes one day. Ten minutes the next. Then 15 minutes. Then go to 15 minutes twice a day and so on, building up time. Keep at it. Keep practicing centering while you're at it. Do it anywhere at all. Don't get discouraged and quit altogether. No matter how short the period, you have at least exerted your will power and reaped some benefit. Your leg muscles were built to hold you up. Use them. Don't leave them hanging there on your locked-up bones like they're paralyzed. If they get tired or quivery, don't give up. Shift weight leg to leg. Dance the box step. Walk in a little circle. Step forward and back again and again. Try not to get discouraged and give up, even if you feel like you're having a nervous breakdown. Take a timeout and sit down. Sit and rest if only for a moment. The feeling **will** pass. It just means your legs are not strong enough – *yet!* If there is no alternative, lock the knees to rest, then unlock them as long as you can. Eventually, you will be spending more time unlocked. Eventually, you will be spending all of your time unlocked.

Every second you spend centering is a victory for you and your body throughout your life. If you keep at it, in time it will become an unnoticed habit. Eventually the victories will come and go with little if any notice. What will be noticeable is that you do not have cellulite.

### Weight loss

With Perfect Posturing, all the muscles of the body, most notably the buttocks and legs, are in a normal state of continuous slight tension or tonus. Using all those large, previously drooping muscles all the time you are standing or walking will burn a lot of calories. That will help keep or get the pounds off. But, it is not a cure-all for obesity. Compare Perfect Posture to the floodgates on a dam. You can open the gates on the dam more but if more water is coming in than they can release, water is going to spill over the top. Perfect Posture may open the comparative caloric gates of the body wider to release, or burn, more calories. But, if more calories are coming in than even Perfect Posturing can release or burn, they are still going to spill over the belt buckle. The only consolation would be that with Perfect Posturing, there would be some tone and proportion to the excess weight – *if* you had the fortitude to carry it all on unlocked knees.

These are some of the more common effects of locking the knees and assuming an unbalanced posture. There are many others but, time and space are money. You and I probably have no more of either to spend on this. Unlock those knees. Practice the progressions and visualizations you'll learn later in the book. Get used to that feeling of balance. Get those legs strong.

# Chapter Three
# What Perfect Posture Can Do
## Part Two:
## The Big Picture

This chapter will illustrate the big picture, or wide angle, of what Perfect Posturing can do. It will follow the development of three individuals, with three different body types, for their entire life. All will start at the age of one or so, when people first begin to stand upright. It will then follow each to age 90, showing the evolving physical changes that occur with each body type. They will all begin as toddlers with illustrations showing the centered way to stand. It's the way a baby stands. It's the way you were designed to stand. Basically, it's the way you should stand your whole life. You should become straighter and more upright as balance and confidence increased with age but, the balancing posture with unlocked knees should be kept for life.

The individual on the inside of the left pages will illustrate an evolution of the centered way to stand. He will always stand with his knees just slightly unlocked. All his points of centering will be consistently kept in proper alignment as indicated by the commandments. He will not accept bent, crooked and soft as "part of the aging process" as the non-centered examples do.

The two on the right-hand pages will follow the progression of two individuals who almost always lock their knees back and "stand up straight." It's the way most are influenced by parents, schools and by example. It's the way most are influenced by culture to stand from birth to death. It's the way most become bent, crooked and soft.

The upper right page illustrations will follow the progression of an individual with above-the-waist creep. The lower-right page illustrations will follow the progression of an individual with below-the-waist creep characteristics.

See if you see anything of yourself, your father, grandfather, or even people around you in any of the examples.

"Getting old" is an expression routinely used when the body falls apart, bulges or bends where you wish it didn't. But, it isn't necessarily so. Make that choice and be the centered, proportioned and toned example on the inside left pages of the chapter. Skip all the exercise besides. Do the best you can. Hover over where you know and feel the center is. Remember to forget rigidity. If you unlock your knees, relax your shoulders and habitually center yourself, your body will fall into place and become toned.

The illustrations will show the basic principles of correct and incorrect body mechanics as they evolve. Through the miracle of illustration, the babies will age to an old man in one chapter. What is not so miraculous is that the individual that keeps his points of center align*ing* will retain the proper body form and tone through his whole life. He will not accept saggy buttocks, saddlebags, potbelly, painful back, cellulite, sore joints or any of the other characteristics of noncentered habits.

## Evolution; the Motion Picture

In the left page sidebars, you'll see an alternate evolution of the same two uncentered individuals from the right hand pages. It will be an evolution toward *becoming* centered. This will be, as they say in the movie business, a "motion picture." It will be opposite to the continued unbalanced postural habits on the right-hand pages. They will stop at 50 and assume a balanced positioning. They will unlock their knees and practice centering habits. They will progress to a centered Perfect Posture over a two year period.

The first illustrations in the left sidebar sequence are the individuals at 50, straight from page 85, with locked knees and all. The second illustrations in the sequence will show them assuming an initial balanced postural positioning. They will have their knees unlocked and points centered as best they can considering their crooked spines. They will not look perfect, but they have to start somewhere. The remaining illustrations will show their evolution to a straighter, balanced and evenly toned Perfect Posture. Flip rapidly through the pages. See the re-adjusting and development of the two 50-year-olds to a centered Perfect Posture. Read the narratives beside the figures to gain some insight into what it might be like to achieve Perfect Posture. The last illustrations at the end of the chapter are what these examples could look like if they centered themselves for an appropriate amount of time. It will be what they could look like from 50-something to the rest of their lives. When you get to the end of the chapter, look at the sidebar and at the corresponding right page images. Which would you rather be?

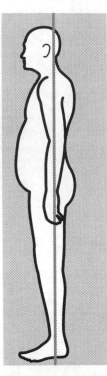

**This is the same 50-year-old from the upper right corner of page 85 standing with the knees locked, spine buckled, and pelvis tilted forward. Creep has occurred mostly above the level of the waist with characteristic swayback, protruding abdomen and slumping shoulders. He will progress to a Perfect Posture in two years.**

When you're one year old you aren't affected by cultural influences. You haven't been introduced to all the cultural nuances, protocols, formalities, proper limits and manners. You've got a clean slate. Not much of a conscience. No real idea of what's right or wrong in one's conduct or motives. You're not troubled by the idea of having acted wrongfully. Not really aware of, or sensitive to anyone's existence, thoughts or surroundings outside of yourself. Nature is your behavioral compass. You do what feels good in thought and action. That would include the way you stand. Directly below and on the right page are the three individuals that will evolve to age ninety years in the course of this chapter.

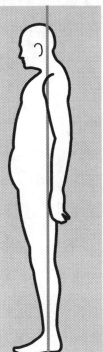

**This is the same 50-year-old from the lower right corner of page 85 standing with knees locked, spine buckled and pelvis tilted forward. Creep has occurred mostly below the level of the waist. Characteristic flat buttocks and backward leaning stance. He will progress to a Perfect Posture in two years.**

### Perfect Posture

The correct way to stand, the way a baby stands. His knees are unlocked and his points of centering are maintained because he hasn't gotten old enough to be influenced by cultural norms. He will stand up straighter as his balance improves but, he will never habitually lock his knees. This example will retain centered posturing his whole life. He will remain toned and proportioned his whole life - front to back, side to side, top to bottom.

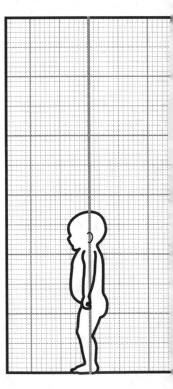

### Above the Waist

This is also the correct way to stand, the way a baby stands. This example will develop creep from the waist up. This type is characterized by a relatively high arch to the low back, pronounced forward arched or hunchbacked upper spine and protrusion of the entire abdomen. No problems yet, of course. He's just a baby.

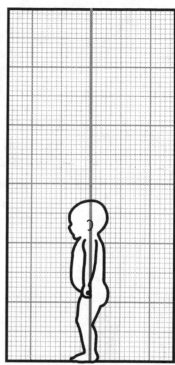

### Below the Waist

Again the correct way to stand and no problems yet. He isn't influenced by culture yet. This example will represent the progression of an individual with creep from the waist down. This type is characterized by relatively flat arch to the low back, flat and tucked-under buttocks, leaning-back stature and potbelly or protrusion in the lower portion of the abdomen.

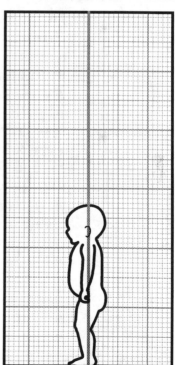

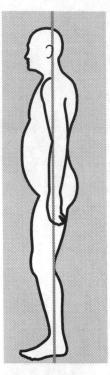

This individual has now unlocked his knees. He's concentrating on his points of center. If he can endure the shaky legs until they're stronger, his feelings of awkwardness and the initial notice of those who know him well, he's on his way.

This is the age when we are at maximum imprintability by most accounts. The individual below has parents who tell him to never lock his knees and to keep his shoulders relaxed. The two to the right (page 75) follow the lead of their parents. They start to "stand up straight" like they're told, like their role models stand, like pictures and statues of their roll models stand.

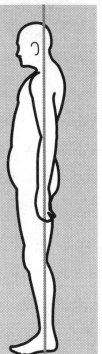

This individual has also now unlocked his knees. He's thinking of his points of centering. His legs and buttocks are quivery with a burning sensation when his knees are unlocked for longer periods. That cranky old woman at work asks why he's "standing there all bendy leggedy." He wonders if this is going to work. Sometimes he has to lock his knees to rest.

### Perfect Posture

Five is the age indoctrination usually starts in earnest. This example will not be indoctrinated, won't become bent and crooked. He won't have parents that tell him to stand up straight and *hold* himself that way. Stresses are equal the majority of the time, front to back, side to side, from top to bottom.

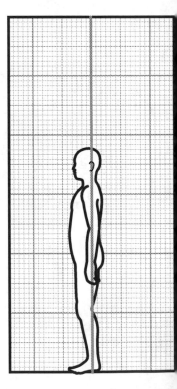

### Above the Waist

Trying to please, this example locks the knees and "stands up straight." He *holds* his shoulders back, like his parents tell him, thus increasing the already over-arched low back. The lower spine is experiencing its first instances of buckling. Stresses are unbalanced the length of the body, but mostly the low back area.

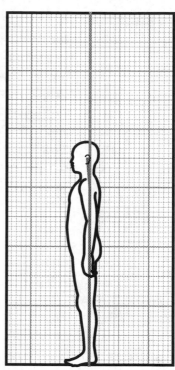

### Below the Waist

Trying to imitate his father or a role model, he too is standing with his knees locked and *holding* his upper body rigid. Not much damage done at this point. His body is still developing. He would lose the buckle in the low back immediately if the knees were unlocked. Stresses would become balanced over the length of the body.

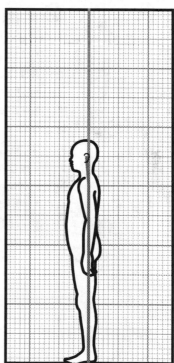

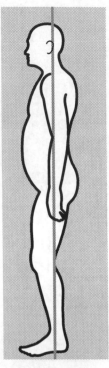

It's been two weeks and it still feels funny standing and walking with slightly bent knees. He's not attracting as much attention as he thought he would. A concerned supervisor asks him if his back is bothering him.

Cultural norms usually have become entrenched at this age. The below example has parents who tell him to unlock his knees and relax his shoulders. They've told him about his points of centering. The instructions are unusual, but won't get him into trouble. In the examples to the right (page 77), the knees are locked. Their parents have told them to "stand up straight and tall with chin up, chest out, stomach in and shoulders back."

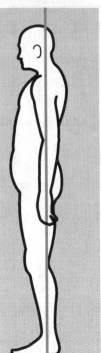

It's been two weeks. His legs get tired and quivery fast. He's unsure if this can be worth it, but he's read the book and it seems to make sense. He's determined to stick it out. He does notice that his back feels better after curling up every night as the book instructed.

## Perfect Posture

Perfect Posturing will be maintained. Knees are unlocked and points of centering vertically aligned. whenever possible. He's on his way to fitness his whole life without exercise. He will maintain a properly proportioned, evenly toned body, front to back, side to side from top to bottom.

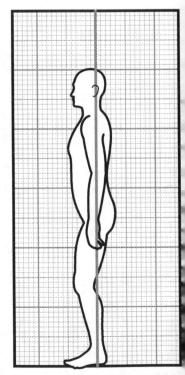

## Above the Waist

This 12-year-old has succumbed to cultural influences and the eventual physical modification that goes with it. He's locking the knees and "standing up straight" as he should. Not much happening yet. Youth is keeping the ravages of unbalanced postural habits at bay. He has a pronounced arch to the low back and a slight hint of slumping shoulders.

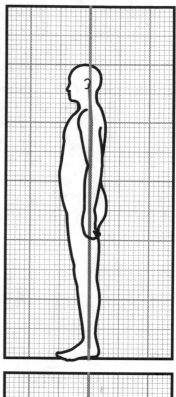

## Below the Waist

This 12-year-old is also doing as he's told. He's trying to "be good." He wants to look and act grown up. He has a slight hint of the buttocks creeping under and leaning back stature when standing. Below-waist creep will become more apparent as he ages. Correction would be almost immediate if Perfect Posture positioning were adopted.

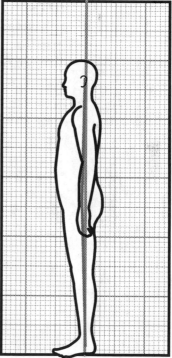

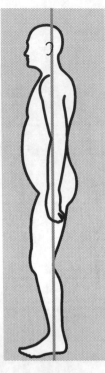

Four weeks of unlocked knees and concentrating on centering points. No one has noticed him practicing centering several times a day. Instead of bending over he crouches to refresh his sense of balance on unlocked knees.

The below example is keeping his points centered, resting the upper body on the legs with the knees unlocked. He's maintaining a natural balance. His shoulders are almost always relaxed. The upper body is *resting* upon, not being *held* above, the pelvis. He is resisting the admonitions to "stand up straight." This would result in unbalanced stresses becoming habitual. Cultural influences in the examples to the right (page 79) have been unconsciously adopted. Stresses are routinely unbalanced along the length of their spines.

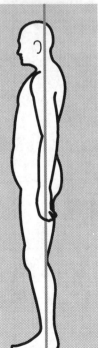

Four weeks of unlocked knees. Practicing centering without notice. Co-workers are used to his new way of standing — no more questions. Legs are so quivery at times he thinks he's having a nervous breakdown. He sits down and the feeling passes.

## Perfect Posture

No changes in postural biomechanics. His body will maintain this form without exercise as long he is alive or changes his postural habits. He is intelligently designing his physical evolution. He's not mindlessly letting culture bend him according to its whim.

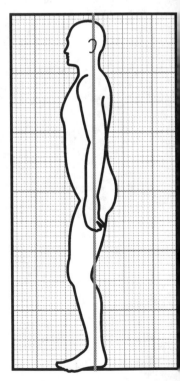

### Above the Waist

No changes in postural habits. Knees solidly locked, shoulders held up straight. His parents and their friends compliment him on how straight and tall he is. He has gotten in the habit of locking his knees back, then standing and resting with his feet spaced widely apart.

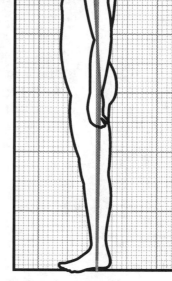

### Below the Waist

This individual, with creep below the waist, is starting to notice the initial characteristic flat bottom and under arched low back. Buttocks are starting to tuck under. Legs are not too weak yet. He could change to a balanced posture and adapt in a few months. He has gotten in the habit of locking his knees back, then standing with his feet close together and parallel. He feels this looks very respectable.

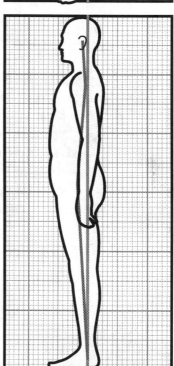

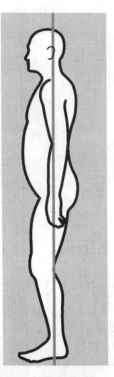

**Above the waist creep adjustment continues. It's been three months. His legs are not so shaky so soon after standing for a while. He thinks he sees a difference, but he's not quite sure. He frequently forgets and lapses into his old way of standing.**

Because the below individual has been following the commandments in the privacy of his own mind and body, his stature remains straight and true. He almost never locks his knees. He's made a habit of keeping his feet the width of the hips and at a 30-degree angle from each other. He doesn't have to go through an uncomfortable process of re-educating his body. Alterations are starting to be noticeable in the two to the right (page 81).

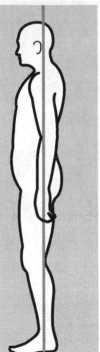

**Below the waist creep adjustment continues. It's been three months. His knees are not so shaky so soon after standing for a while. He stands the old way sometimes to rest when he can't sit down. He tries to do so only as last resort.**

### Perfect Posture

He is still occasionally admonished by superiors or authority figures to sit up straight when he slouches too far in a straight backed chair. He sits up out of respect or deference.

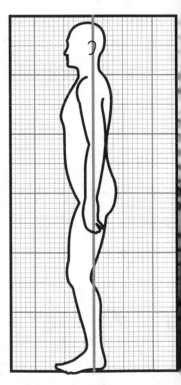

## Above the Waist

This individual is doing all the right things. He has stood up straight just as he's been told he should. Despite his best intentions, he's had to start painful, repetitious exercises to maintain the appearance of fitness. His slumping shoulders are becoming noticeable. The full-length protruding belly is starting to annoy him. It's taking more and more sit-ups to keep it flat. Better start eating right.

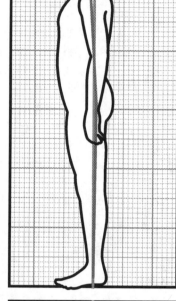

## Below the Waist

Alteration, drift, creep, deformity, getting old, or whatever you want to call it, is getting ramped up. The buttocks are really starting to tuck under. He envies people with round contoured buttocks. He has been lifting weights and doing sit-ups. The deep knee bends with the weight on his shoulders make his hips sore but, he feels it's the price you pay for fitness. He's buff but he wishes he didn't have a flat bottom and a sort of leaning-back stature.

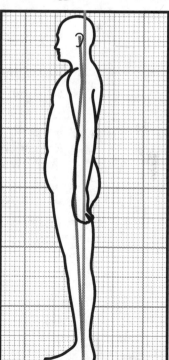

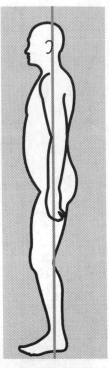

**It's been six months. He's getting a little impatient. He looks in a mirror and pushes his nose firmly to the side for one full minute, then lets it go. It takes a long time for the nose to return to its natural position. He reflects on the years pushing his spine out of shape. He shrugs and thinks: takes time.**

What is perfect one moment will not be the next, depending on outside influence or observation of the individual. Do not become stiff or rigid. Know where perfection lies but, don't expect to *hold* it like a chunk of stone. "Hunka", the name for a Lakota ceremony that means "to forever move," should be kept in mind. Forever move. Hover in, out and around your center. Life is fluid. You should be too.

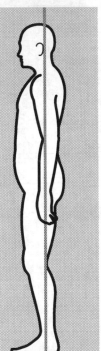

**It's been six months with the knees mostly unlocked. He wonders if he can really see some progress. His legs are getting noticeably stronger, less quivery. He finds himself standing in the old way at times. He quickly unlocks the knees and centers himself.**

### Perfect Posture

He still has a youthful appearance. He's always mindful to keep his shoulders, hips and anklebones vertical to each other. But, he's not obsessive about it. He thinks about it when standing in lines. He keeps his weight shifting foot to foot, dances the box step. He doesn't get too far away from the centering points, for too long, when fidgeting from leg to leg.

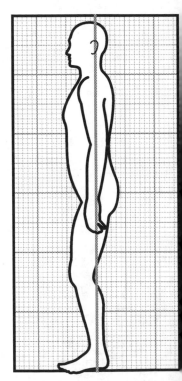

### Above the Waist

Even with exercise, he can't seem to get totally rid of his protruding belly. He has had to slow down on sit-ups and weightlifting due to a sore back. His back and shoulders are slumped more and more despite a conscious effort to hold them straight.

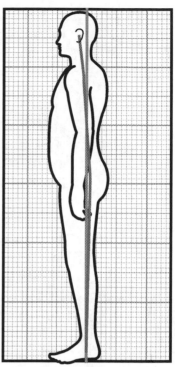

### Below the Waist

His shoulders do not slump forward as much as the above individual because he has unconsciously curled his buttocks under. This lessens the arch and tension in the buckled low back. He appears to be leaning back when he talks to someone. This is because the area below the waist has moved forward of the shoulders.

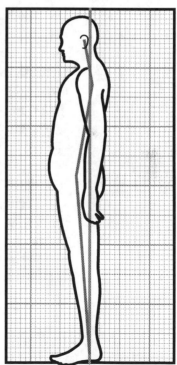

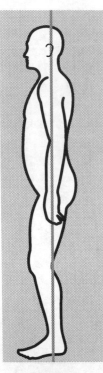

It's been nine months. He's thinking about cultural influences frequently. He's practicing progression #1 every night at bedtime. He's sleeping better. His sore, stiff low back is better. Frequently he practices a crouch to refresh his sense of equilibrium. It occurred to him that his left knee doesn't pop and get sore anymore when he's stuck in traffic and has to shift gears a lot.

When you stand according to the commandments, the backbones naturally form the pitch and angle they were created for. The push of the body up and the pull of gravity down are then balanced throughout the body and its joints. If they are not balanced, there will be unequal push or pull on muscles, ligaments and joints. Stresses will be unequal with continuous strain front to back or side to side. Things can't help but go "out of shape" or "fall apart."

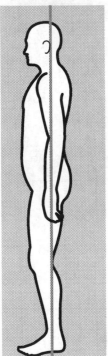

Nine months. He practices crouching whenever he can to re-educate his body parts to the *feel* for the balanced position. He's surprised his hips feel better, not worse, with all the practice. He maintains position #1 religiously for 15 minutes before going to sleep. He can't believe how good his back feels.

## Perfect Posture

He is a little embarrassed when people ask how he stays in shape. They tell him how good he looks. He smiles and thinks it must be all that beer. A niece who's around for a family reunion tells him he hasn't changed since he was in San Diego 25 years ago.

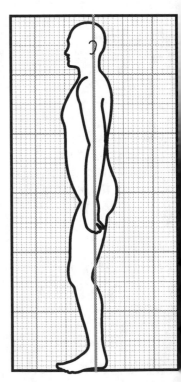

### Above the Waist

He has gotten somewhat used to the idea of middle age. He's toned down versions of exercise. He has a definite slouch to his shoulders. No more sit-ups due to back pain. He may have to see the doctor and consider back surgery again. He still has the habit of standing with his feet too far apart and at a wide angle to each other.

An alternative sequence of this individual, starting on page 72, shows what would hapen if he chose Perfect Posture positioning at this age.

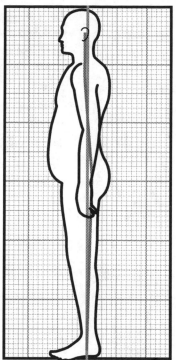

### Below the Waist

His buttocks seem to be sagging more and more. He consciously curls his buttocks under to relieve low-back discomfort. He still has the habit of standing with his feet close together and parallel to each other. He still thinks it makes him look respectable.

An alternative sequence of this individual, starting on page 72, shows what would happen if he chose Perfect Posture positioning at this age.

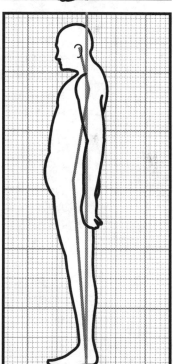

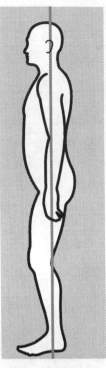

One year with knees unlocked a lot of the time now. He's lost 20 pounds. He finds it easier to stand for extended periods without quivery legs. He's gotten in the habit of shifting weight from leg to leg in smooth, flowing motion. He sits down when necessary.

The below individual who practices the principles of Perfect Posture still has a square, straight frame. He has always maintained a conscious effort to keep his points centered and his knees unlocked. Most of the time it's automatic and no one even knows he does anything in particular to stay in shape. It's just that when he's had a moment, he has centered. Whether walking or standing, just a moment to practice. When he sits, he reclines whenever possible.

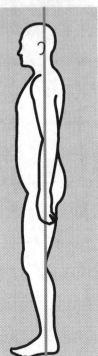

One year of trying to maintain unlocked knees. He's managing to keep them unlocked most of the time now. He can't believe he doesn't have the flat buttocks and backward leaning posture like his father. And he thought it was unavoidable – genetically predestined. It was tough getting used to unlocked knees though.

## Perfect Posture

He is still going strong with a youthful appearance at 60. His body still maintains its youthful contours. He still disdains repetitious, strenuous exercise. He can still compete with his 30-year-old son in tennis. His ankles, knees and hips are still in good shape because he's always kept them properly aligned.

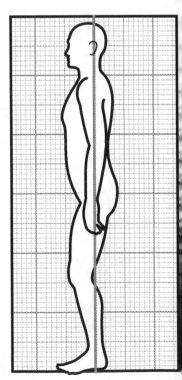

## Above the Waist

He finally got that back surgery so that doesn't hurt. It's stiff but at least it doesn't hurt. He still has the sore knees though. His habit of standing with his feet too far apart has had unbalanced compression effects and chronically inflamed the outside of the knees and top part of the hip joints.

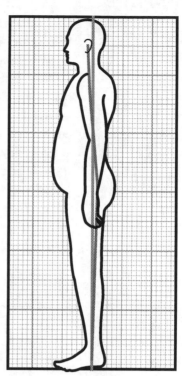

## Below the Waist

His buttocks continue tucking under and his upper body seems to lean back more and more. His hips are always sore because of chronically standing with his feet too close together. Couple this with the weight on the backside of the hip joint from always tucking it under. Doctor calls it arthritis. He may have to consider a hip replacement in the near future. Exercise has little appeal.

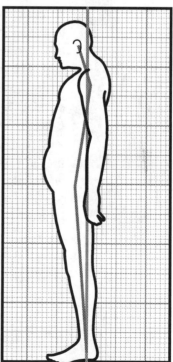

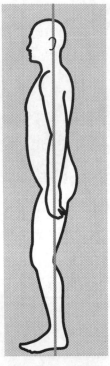

It's been a year and a half. He still relapses to the old way of standing at times – mostly mornings. He always has centering on his mind, whether standing or walking. It's become a habit, almost without thinking now because he's so happy with how he looks.

# Seventy Years Old

It's not hard to say which commandment is most important: Never lock the knees. But, just one commandment not adhered to will throw a whole system out of whack. It will radiate unbalanced stresses to other parts of the body. The individual below has always kept his points of center in the back of his mind. He's seldom locked his knees so his legs aren't weak. He still catches himself locking them but. overall. he's been pretty good about it. It shows. The two on the right (page 89) have not. They have weak legs, sore stiff knees and hips.

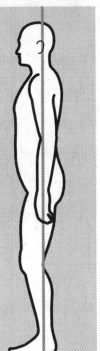

It's been a year and a half. This is the body he knew he could have. And to think it was done without exercise. Everything is falling into place. He's toned and proportioned – the way he should be. He has to sit down to rest his legs sometimes, but he had to do that before, too.

## Perfect Posture

Seventy something and still has straight, square frame. That same niece sees him and asks if he is ever going to get old. His movements are still quick and agile. He is going on a mountain hike next week. Better prepare. Get plenty of beer, hotdogs and S'mores.

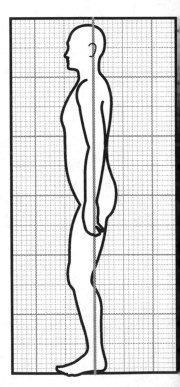

### Above the Waist

He's seventy now and has chronic sore knees. He has trouble stooping and getting back up. His shoulders are highly slouched. He takes a daily walk around the park. It's a nice, level terrain. He has trouble walking up stairs because of arthritic knees, especially the left one. He has given up on exercise.

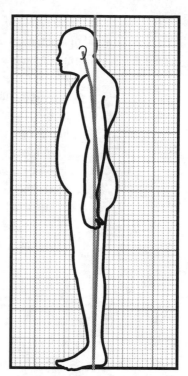

### Below the Waist

His buttocks continue to tuck. They're flat, wrinkled and soft. He walks with a cane. He still has the habit of standing with his feet too close together. His hips are always sore. Doctor diagnoses arthritis and informs him he may do well to get the right one replaced. He also has occasional pain in the very low back, upper buttocks area. It radiates down his right leg at times.

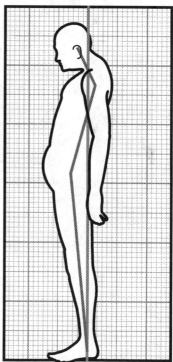

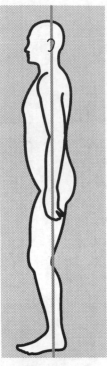

One year and nine months. He's comfortable with an unlocked posture. He does it without thinking most of the time. An old woman at work says "you have a nice walk." He's proportioned and evenly toned. All from force of habit. Who would have thought?

The below individual has remained as close to his center as he could and hovered around it. At an early age he got used to the positional impressions, the *feel* of balance, so it became automatic. His legs and buttocks, and belly are still toned, proportioned and strong. His joints are healthy. The examples to the right (page 91) have "gotten old" with stooped, crooked, bulging postures, and movement that is slow and guarded.

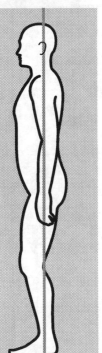

One year and nine months. His chest, shoulders, abdomen, buttocks and legs are all smooth, toned and proportioned in a balanced resting tonus. All done with the convenient use of mind and body. Fitness without exercise. What a concept!

## Perfect Posture

He's still a little embarrassed that he doesn't exercise when people ask how he does it. When he says body "mechanics or structural hygiene", a puzzled look is the response. But he has given up on trying to explain it in passing conversation. Though not really complicated, it's difficult to explain quickly.

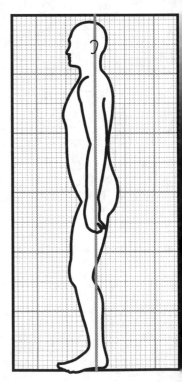

### Above the Waist

He is now bent and crooked. Crouching is out of the question without help. Exercise consists of rolling his shoulders in a circle or lifting a foot while sitting in a chair. He walks down the block to the store to get out of the house daily. He has to decide if the benefits of total left knee replacement are worth it at his age.

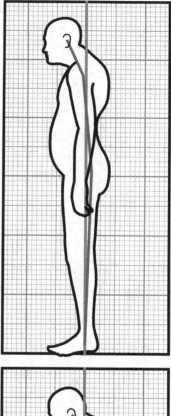

### Below the Waist

Even with below-waist creep taking the pressure off the low back, the upper back has bent forward trying to maintain a balanced orientation. Otherwise he would fall down backwards. He carries an alarm to summon help if he should fall to the floor. He's afraid he couldn't get up by himself. He got the right hip replaced last year. He has to decide whether to do the other one at his age.

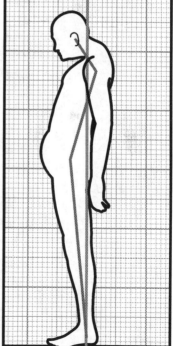

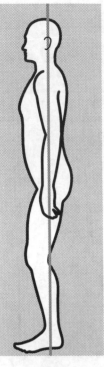

Two years. He ran into a friend he hadn't seen in six years. The friend didn't recognize him at first and looked puzzled, then realized who he was and looked puzzled again. The friend says he looks different and wants to know what exercises he's been doing. He's now confident anyone could correct poor posture.

This is where the illustrations end. The evolution has been demonstrated. Is becoming bent and crooked part of the aging process? The below individual knows this isn't so. He knows anyone could look like this at 90. He knows of no research evidence to indicate that posture has to worsen with age. He knows poor posture develops as you age but is not part of the aging process. For the individuals on the right (page 93), walking is a chore. Their bodies are bent and crooked, like a spring that's been unbalanced for a long time. Everyone has to wait for them whenever they walk somewhere because their movements are slow and guarded. They never knew poor posture could be corrected.

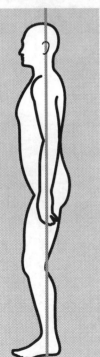

Two years. He happens into an old friend he hasn't seen in years. The friend says he looks different and it's not just the weight loss. His friend wants to know what exercise program he uses. He smiles and says it's difficult to explain in five words or less. He tells the friend to read the book. He's now confident he can maintain Perfect Posture the rest of his life.

## Perfect Posture

He's still able to practice centering by crouching. This is because he never locked his knees, ruining them and his hips. His leg muscles have never weakened from lack of use. If an individual should live this long, this is how he would look routinely using balanced body mechanics and keeping his knees unlocked.

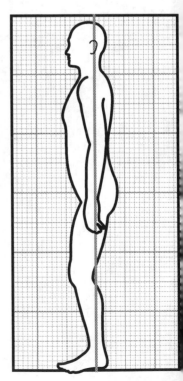

### Above the Waist

The hunchback and slouching shoulders are severe. If an individual should live this long, this is how he would look using culturally indoctrinated body mechanics and having fully developed above-the-waist creep. Note, the other version of this same individual in the left page sidebar. That is what he could have looked like now if he had adopted proper habits at 50. Which would you rather be?

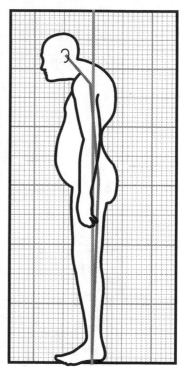

### Below the Waist

He's worried about falling because his joints are stiff and his leg muscles are too weak for him to get up by himself. He never really recovered from the second hip replacement. If an individual should live this long, this is how he might look with fully developed below-the-waist creep. Note, the other version of this same individual in the left page sidebar. That is what he could have looked like now if he had adopted proper habits at 50. Which would you rather be?

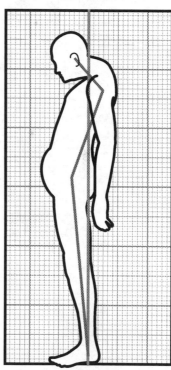

# Chapter Four
# How To Get Perfect Posture

## Part One:
## Progressing to an Ideal

By now, you know that standing with your knees locked to the rear is the most widespread and dominant cause of poor posture. The immediate effect is a buckled waist level spine and forward tipped pelvis. These are the chief effects that give rise to the two basic types of creep. From the combinations of these two types of creep arise the countless varieties of physical alteration called poor posture or the aging process. Most people in our culture and many others are affected with them to some degree. Trying to fix all these different problems separately is just too complicated.

What you need to do then, is get to the root of the problems. Stop the process before it gets complicated. Keep those knees unlocked so that the low back can stretch out and develop a balanced curvature with proper pitch, angle and spacing. Then the spine, both above and below the waist, can respond accordingly and develop a balanced curvature with proper pitch, angle and spacing. Then you won't have all those different problems to fix. You won't have all those different machines to buy, exercises to do or procedures to endure that really don't solve the problems anyway .

Unlocking the knees can be done as quickly and easily as snapping the fingers. So you might as well take care of that right now. **Unlock those knees and keep them unlocked!**

Now that that's taken care of, you can concentrate on the time-consuming adjustments. Number one is getting that waist-level spine unbuckled and the pelvis leveled. Number two is patiently getting the legs strong enough to hold you for reasonable amounts of time. This may be more difficult than you think. Number three is getting used to the new sense of your body's position as felt from within. Becoming a new you, inside and out, takes courage. You may think you look as funny as you feel. Handling the initial attention, a different way of standing and walking draws can be difficult. This might be the hardest.

The progressions in this chapter are mostly meant to get at those chief effects of locking the knees: that buckled back and tilted pelvis. I call them progressions because, in all likelihood, you will be advancing from an initial position to an ideal. They will help stretch the low back so it can more quickly lose some of that buckle and level the pelvis. Be careful with the words "more quickly." Don't get too excited and set yourself up for discouragement. Be realistic. You have to bend some of the arch out of that stiff, thick, waist-level back. This takes time. It takes time to bend the thick, muscular area around the sacroiliac to a more level position. It takes time to strengthen the legs and buttocks. It takes time to get used to the new messages your muscles, tendons and joints are sending you about your body's position. It takes time for the chest level spine to uncreep and assume its more straightened position. It takes time to develop the muscle balance strength to comfortably hold all these parts in equilibrium. Did I mention this process takes time? We're talking about hard tissues: ligaments and cartilage. Not just muscles. Keep at it. Don't give up, no matter how little or great your advancement. Enter a new era in your life.

The reason I'm running this "takes time" business into the ground is because I want you to firmly understand you should not get impatient, discouraged and quit. Go slow with these progressions. Going too fast can cause injury. If you feel pain, stop what you're doing, return to a previous, less-advanced form of a progression. Pain equals damage. Slow down; give it a rest and decrease the intensity of what you're doing. Keep it slow, moderate and consistent, or, just don't bother with them at all. Without these positional progressions, the spine would still return to the proper curvature if the centering commandments are internalized. It would just take longer and you wouldn't be flexible. You would be stiff, but stiff in the properly proportioned, balanced and evenly toned form – front to back, side to side, from top to bottom. Perfect Posturing is a way of life. It's not the latest crash program you're going to see results with immediately. It's not a six-minute, six-hour, six-day, six-week, six-month or even six-year program. It's a program for life.

If you have a bad or injured back, you may have to modify these progressions to apply the least amount of strain as possible. Modify them about any way you want. **Flexibility and Reshaping** are the key words. Place pillows - as will be shown - to relieve pressure or strain in any of the horizontal progressions. If something hurts, stop what you're doing. Wait a day or two, and start again with a less strenuous level of the progression. Consult a qualified professional to be sure you don't have a pre-existing condition that could contradict or cause a need to modify any of these positions.

The following positional progressions can be used to speed up the process to Perfect Posture and can be used to varying degrees of extremity, duration and frequency. Remember: you are not building up anything. You are stretching ligaments and re-forming cartilage so you can feel comfortable standing in an anatomically balanced manner. You are bending the stiff low back in the opposite direction it has been buckled.

Position one is a preparation to perform position number two. This position is one of the best, and least dangerous, of the progressions. As with all, you should still proceed with caution to avoid injury. As with all, jerking or pulling can strain muscles, pull ligaments, rupture discs or even crush a vertebra. These are progressions to an ideal. Some may be able to assume the ideal positions immediately. Some others may take a considerable amount of time to comfortably reach the ideal. Some may never reach, or want to reach, the ideal. Don't worry. The ideal in any of these positions is not essential for attaining Perfect Posture anyway.

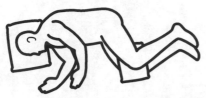

**Image 6.01**
**Initial position while laying on side.**

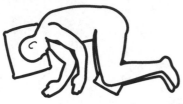

**Image 6.02**
**Mid position of curl.**

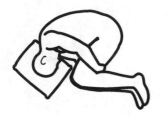

**Image 6.03**
**Completed fetal position.**

## Horizontal Progressions

### Progression one: beginning unbuckling

This is how you do it, with some do's and don'ts. While lying on your side in bed, ease your nose toward your knees as much as you comfortably can. Put a pillow under your head and point your nose straight ahead. Try to keep your shoulders vertical to each other. Keep your knees vertical to each other. Put a pillow between them. [Image 6.01] Gradually work up to the position of nose to knees. If you must pull on your knees, pull them toward your nose from the back of the knees. Pulling from the front puts pressure on your low back. If you have a touchy or sore back, you can injure yourself and slow your progress. No jerking or straining!

This would be the mid position. It's about the normal for most people at first. [Image 6.02]

The end result is sometimes called the fetal position. Essentially, you're curling up into a ball. In this position your back is in a natural position of perfect traction. Not stretched too much, not stretched too little. It's just right. If you do this for 15 minutes every night for a year, that will equal approximately 91 hours. A sizable amount of time = a sizable amount of progress.

The ideal is when you can maintain the nose to knees position for an hour without discomfort. [Image 6.03] Your back will be stretched enough to feel comfortable in the centered, standing position indefinitely. Getting to this position can take minutes, days, weeks, or even years depending on your pre-existing condition and time spent stretching. Take it slow. Straining is counter productive.

If you have large hips and it seems uncomfortable in your midsection, put a pillow under there. The whole purpose is to get your low back flexible. Variation doesn't matter. If you want it to be forehead-to-knees, it's all right. Arm placement isn't a big issue. Just so you feel comfortable and you can stretch the low back without it becoming painful. Also you may be pleasantly surprised to find you sleep better and wake up feeling better if you practice this progression for 15 minutes every night before falling asleep.

### Progression two: intermediate unbuckling

Progression #2 is also a series of progressions toward an ideal. It is not necessary to attain the ideal in this progression or any other to obtain a positive effect or Perfect Posture. So don't get too worked up about this flexibility business. It's necessary only if you want to speed the process. When you can assume the fetal position for an hour without discomfort in position #1, you can start on stretching the low back and spine even more.

Remember, no sweating, turning red, straining, jerking or heavy breathing required. These are also thinking maneuvers. You're working toward feeling and knowing inside yourself **when** the body is correctly positioned.

This is how you do this one. [Image 6.04]

Lay on your back on a soft surface such as a carpet, mat or even your bed. With both knees bent to a 45-degree angle, start propping your head and shoulders up with pillows while doing the same with your buttocks. [A] Continue propping until you've got the small of your back comfortably pressed onto the surface. Rest, and let your low back stretch. [B] When your low back is pressed into the bed or floor without effort, you can start removing pillows. Keep progressing to fewer and fewer pillows while lowering your legs. When you can keep your low back pressed into the carpet or mat with little to no effort and just a rolled-up bath towel under your knees, you've reached the ideal. [C] Feel free to keep a pillow under your head for comfort. This position is to give your body an approximate feel for where your body should be when you're standing. This is where the progression should get to - ideal position #2.

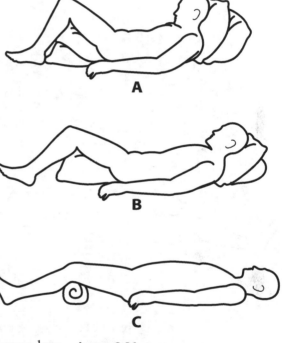

**Image 6.04**
**Progression of stretch:**
( A ) Lots of pillows.
( B ) Fewer pillows.
( C ) No pillows, just a towel under the knees.

## Advanced progression #2

Here is a further step to strengthen and shorten those belly muscles to help hold the pelvis level. This will also help straighten the buckled spine and develop muscle balance strength at the waist level. This step almost resembles that dirty word "exercise." I was tempted to censor this step. Use it cautiously and with mild exertion. [Image 6.05]

Lay in the progression # 2 at any stage of advancement. Whatever it takes to barely unlock the knees and keep the legs relaxed. This will, in turn, unlock the pelvis and make it easier to get the low back unbuckled and flat on the surface. Keep the feet the width of the hips and relaxed. Hands relaxed at your sides. Inhale normally but, when you exhale, purse your lips in order to restrict the flow of air from your lungs. Push with your stomach muscles to force the air out. Purse lips as much as you're comfortable with to get the air expelled. The more you purse your lips, the harder to expel the air, the more you strengthen your abdomen. No need to go to extremes to the point of making yourself dizzy and injuring yourself with a strained muscle or worse. Just purse your lips and tense the abdomen comfortably to exhale. You are strengthening the abdominal muscles right at the balanced spot you'll need to feel comfortable in your new standing position.

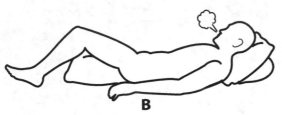

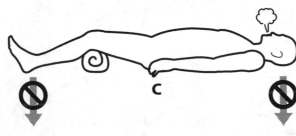

**Image 6.05 Controlled breathing.**

You're pulling the buckle out of your spine. You'll feel your pelvis curl under and tilt toward the back. Take it slow, with minimal exertion. If it makes you too sore, then just don't do it. You'll reach the objective eventually without it.

**Warning:** If you're sore the next day, stop exerting so much. Take it easy!

**Note**: Don't ever push down on the surface with your head or heels.

Another way of initially starting these progressions is with a papasan chair. [Image 6.06] It's a good, cheap investment and it's the natural form for your resting back. A recliner could also be used. Then, you could keep using them all the time so you could continue healthy sitting habits and keep the back properly stretched. Be creative. The result you're working toward is a back that is flexible enough to assume proper curvature in the standing position — a back that is not stiffly formed in the buckled position. The methods of achieving it are infinite. Just take it slow. Don't hurt yourself and get discouraged.

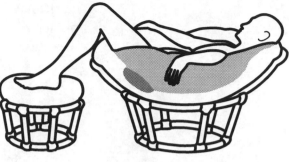

**Image 6.06**
**Papasan chair. No need to stay fully reclined. 120° is fine.**

## Progression three: advanced unbuckling

It's important that you not proceed aggressively with this progression. This one is easy to overdo. Wait until you are comfortable with #1 and #2.

Lay on your back on the same surface you've been using. Roll over backwards. Gently roll your feet over your head, as far as you can comfortably do. Progress until you can touch your knees to your shoulders (ideal position # 3). Most cannot come close to this. Just do the best you can and don't strain or hurt yourself. Don't hold the position too long. You'll get dizzy, or worse, injure your back by doing the correct thing too hard and fast. [Image 6.07]

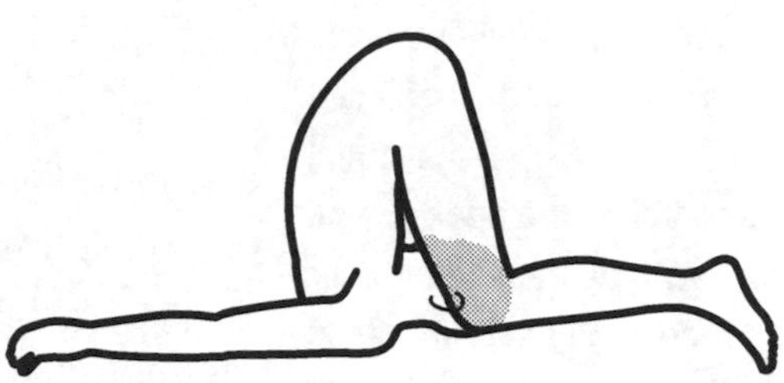

**Image 6.07**
**Do this on an empty stomach so it's not so hard to breath.**

Here's another way of doing these types of stretches. Get one of those big exercise balls at the sporting goods store. Lay on your stomach on it. Lay on your stomach on it and roll back and forth. [Image 6.08] Getting the picture?

**Flexibility and Reshaping** that lumbar spine to an unbuckled form is the picture.

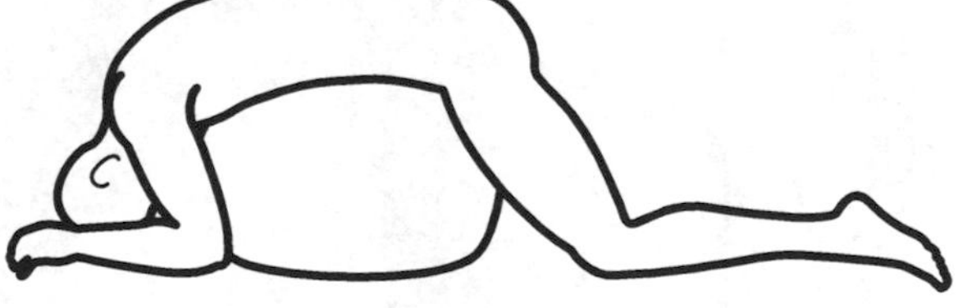

**Image 6.08**
**Using exercise ball.**

It may seem these progressions should only be needed for the clearly buckled low back characteristics of above-the-waist creep. In above-the-waist creep the spine, above the L1 vertebrae, moves forward in a long sweeping curve. You have nineteen vertebras above it to absorb tension from the posterior lumbar spine. Thus the L1, L2 and L3 vertebra don't lose much buckle. This leaves an arch obvious to the eye.

But, they are also needed for the apparently unbuckled, or flat, low back characteristic of below-the-waist creep. The below series of diagrams illustrates why this is so. The shaded part of the illustration will not change. The outline portion of the diagram will move, demonstrating why these progressions are still needed for an unbuckled appearing low back. The first diagram represents the profile of a balanced, properly pitched and angles lumbar spine [A]. The next diagram shows an initial buckled back [B]. In below the waist creep the low back appears unbuckled, or flat, to the eye [C]. It appears flat because the area below the apex only has three movable parts to absorb tension. They creep forward as a nearly straight, rigid unit. But the part of the buckle above the apex is still there – not so obvious to the eye. That part of the buckle has to go. These progressions will do this. When they do, the L1, L2 and L3 vertebras will unbuckle. The L4, L5 vertebrae and sacrum will move back to their natural, more posterior, position [D].

**Image 6.09**
[A] Shaded, outlined profile of balanced properly pitched and angled lumbar spine.
[B] Outline of buckled low back. Shading remains in the balanced position.

[C] The area below the apex creeps forward with decreased anterior pitch and increased posterior pitch.

[D] With progression #1 the L1, L2, and L3 vertebrae have lost the buckle. Consequently the L4, L5 and sacral vertebrae have responded moving posteriorly. The lumbar vertebrae are again properly balanced, pitched and angled.

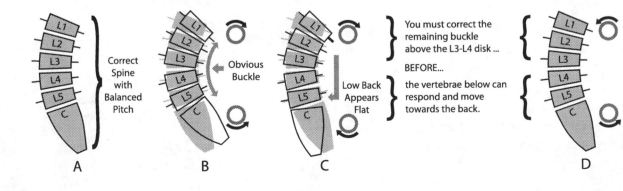

## Vertical Progressions

### Crouching for rest, flexibility, reshaping, strength and balance kinesthesia

The crouch, squat or deep-knee bend is good for at least 5 things when it comes to Perfect Posturing body mechanics. It's the single most valuable of the how to "get it" and "keep it" activities you can do. If you decide on one thing to do to get and keep Perfect Posture, this would be it.

If you get used to it, in the fully crouched position, it's almost as good as sitting down to take a rest. Don't stay in the fully crouched position too long until you're used to it. This can strain your back and make you feel you're doing something wrong. It's not wrong, you're just being too aggressive. You're doing too much, too fast for your stiff back to comfortably stretch and reshape itself.

Crouching strengthens the buttocks and legs so you can feel comfortable standing with unlocked knees. Crouching is the most important progression for developing kinesthesia, that is, your sensations of bodily motion and position as you move. It will help you learn how you feel when your posture is balanced, centered, and symmetrical. Frequent crouching gives a familiarity to your consciousness of where this position is.

> **Kinesthesia is also called muscle sense.**

Most people stop crouching as soon as they're indoctrinated into the socially acceptable, customary way of standing. They bend over. In some other cultures crouching is common. Therefore their heel ligaments aren't shortened. Their knees aren't stiff and don't pop. Their thighs aren't weak, backs aren't compressed, and their balance isn't poor from lack of practice. Don't get too repetitious. In cultures where crouching is a way of life no one does 25 deep-knee bends in a row. It's not how many you can do that you're concerned with in this progression. It's the sense of balance and physical position you're concerned with internalizing. Do one, at the most two or three, just about anytime, anywhere you are.

### Doing the crouch

Go as slowly as you can so you can get a good feel for your kinesthetic impressions. Get two sawhorses, pieces of furniture, a friend or two. Use anything to get you started if your legs are weak. Don't wear shoes, but if you must, as low of heels as possible. If you can't keep your balance in the lowest position, put your heels on a 2-by-4, 4-by-4 or even taller artifact, if you wish. Work your way down to a 1-by-4, then the flat surface for the ideal when you've got your back stretched out. You can keep your hands extended for balance. Ideally you would want to progress to keeping them on your hips or at your sides. Then, eventually, you could crouch and use them for something besides balancing. But that's an intense balance few would care to achieve and totally unnecessary. The Perfect Posture can be obtained by simply remembering your points of center and maintaining them.

**Image 6.10**

**The stages of achieving a squat or crouch position.**

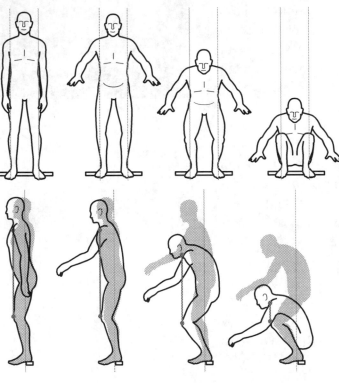

Here's the process. Stand with your knees unlocked and shoulders relaxed (as you of course always do now). Have all points centered as best you can according to the commandments. Immediately before you start your descent, move the shoulders forward to where they're vertical to the front of the knees. Incidentally, this is also the position your shoulders should be at when starting and during walking.

Go all the way down until you hit bottom, with your shoulders or chest on your knees. Keep the knees the width of the hips and second toes. Keep your back relaxed as best you can throughout the process. Remain in this position for a short moment or as long as is comfortable. Let the back relax and stretch. Don't stay in the descended position so long it hurts to straighten up. If your knees pop, or are sore, lubricate them as shown on the following progression.

Start the ascent. Try not to use your back muscles to get you up. Rock yourself forward or back a little to gain your balance and find your center. Up you go using only your leg muscles.

As you begin to rise up, remember to keep the shoulders relaxed, directly above the front of the knees. Try to not use your back muscles to maintain balance. This is hard to do. Just do the best you can. It's an ideal you may not reach and is unnecessary. Just get used to balancing your upper body on your legs as best you can to develop your natural poise. It will take some time. You'll get better and better.

Midway up is the most difficult for most people. Due to unbalanced habits and lack of use, the muscles of the legs have weakened. The muscles of the back and a jerking movement are frequently used to get over this hump. Resist this. As you gain strength and balance, the spot where you needed to pull yourself up with something, those sawhorses, the friendly hand, the jerk of the arms, will not be needed. It will be one smooth operation as slow or fast as you choose. No hump.

Keep the front of the shoulders vertical to the front of the knees throughout the ascent. When you get to the almost standing straight position, stop for a short moment while keeping your shoulders vertical to the front of the knees. Now, position them above your hipbone, dead center above your anklebone. Center your head. Keep the knees unlocked. You are in your new standing position. Concentrate on the feeling.

It will feel odd at first. The worse your habits have been, the

**Image 6.11**
**The stages of ascending from a squat or crouch position. You will find you don't need as much support under the heel when your back is streched out.**

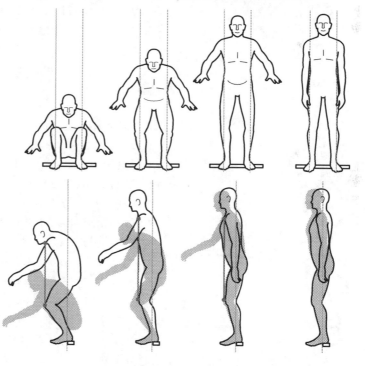

funnier it will feel. Keep practicing in a relaxed, consistent manner. You'll get used to it. Your body will have, or get, its proper and evenly toned form.

You may field some remarks about the way you are standing from people who know you well or are around you on a daily basis. But like a new tattoo or style of dress, they will get used to it and the comments will cease.

### Oiling the knee

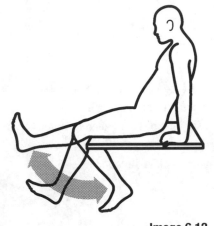

**Image 6.12**
**Oiling the knee.**

You may have knees that are stiff, sore or pop when you crouch. Take those two sawhorses you were using to help you up while crouching and put a piece of plywood over them. Weren't using any for balancing? Get a couple anyway. You can build something when you're not oiling your knee. Sit on the plywood and let one lower leg swing back and forth. Keep it loose or limp. Just let it swing. First swing one for a number of repetitions and then the other. If your knee feels uncomfortable, move further back or forward on the plywood. Reduce the arch of the swing. As you become comfortable, progressively lengthen the arch of the swing. Try a couple of crouches before and after doing the swings. You'll be surprised how much better your knees feel after oiling. [Image 6.12]

### The standing stretch

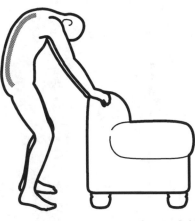

**Image 6.13**
**Standing stretched with support.**

As always, be sure your second toes are directly below the outside of the hips from the front view. Stand at a counter or other sturdy object. Stretch your buttocks and your head forward. The further you can curl the buttocks, the more you are approaching a natural curvature to the back and the more comfortable you will feel standing in a centered posture. Each time you stretch exhale, releasing the resistance of the inflated lungs on your abdomen. Remember, don't go too fast or strain. It can cause injury and destroy your resolve to continue onward. No pain, no gain is not the catch phrase for this system. As with all of the vertical exercises, it can be done most anywhere: Bathroom, desk, telephone pole, telephone booth, almost anywhere including the kitchen sink. [Image 6.13]

Duration and consistency is the key. The more time you spend, or have spent, in unbalanced positions in your life, the more time you'll have to spend doing progressions. Use these or think of your own. Increased flexibility, leg strength and awareness of bodily position are the desired results. The possible methods for getting the desired results are infinite.

# Chapter Five

# How to Keep Perfect Posture

## Part One:
## Practicing Perfect Posture
## Through Visualizations

### Practice Perfect Posture Through Visualizations

Whether standing with knees locked or unlocked, standing requires some effort. As long as you're going to be doing it, do it in a way that's beneficial. This chapter will give you some ways to think about, and practice standing and walking, so it's beneficial.

Outside influences or activities are continuously causing an unbalanced body. A continuous counter-effort must be maintained to keep the body balanced. Don't get lazy, lock your knees and stop this process. It will be left to the bones, joints and ligaments to keep you rigidly locked upright. You'll start to damage them immediately. You'll start to weaken muscles immediately. Your muscles in your legs were built to hold you up. Use them. Get them strong like they're supposed to be.

Getting used to a centered body might be easier for you if you have some visual associations to identify with. This would give you a mental picture to practice balancing gravity on your central axis. This chapter will describe different activities and situations so, throughout the day, you can visualize them and try to move in the manner required for those activities.

Always remember, your body is not static. You should always stand as if the surface is unstable. If you become static or try to hold these visualization positions, you will feel exceedingly unnatural and rigid. The object of these visualizations is to make you aware of this so that a continual subtle movement is unconscious. Just let your natural symmetries find their groove. Frequent practice will make it

automatic and unnoticeable in everyday life when movement is accelerated and unconscious. It will be as natural to you as your old way of standing and moving. Practice visualizations just about anywhere, if you use a moderated version.
No need to make a spectacle of yourself.

You could center your head during a pause at your desk. Every time you go to the bathroom you could practice a walking visualization, to get accustomed to the feeling of being centered and gain the benefits of Perfect Posturing. Keep your mind open. You don't have to use these visualizations. Since you have learned the points of centering, you'll be able to think of your own variations on these themes.

While doing any of these visualization positionings, keep the commandments you've learned and are trying to get accustomed to in the back of your mind.

Becoming comfortable with having unlocked knees may be the most difficult single point of this system for you. The habit of standing with the knees locked has been imprinted in most so intensely, for so long, that it feels extremely awkward to stand correctly. From verbal indoctrination, to visual example, to the chairs we sit in, we are immersed from the time we're born into the culture of concretized images of how we should look. No small wonder this new way of standing feels funny.

This is repetitious, but it must be done to help stop you from identifying with the idea that the deformities resultant to these cultural influences are inevitable. You *can* contour the body to the tight, proportioned, smooth machine it was meant to be – front to back, side to side from top to bottom. You can keep it that way for the rest of your life. **Without exercise.**

If you're looking to get buff or muscle-bound, Perfect Posture is not about that. You'll have to do that on your own. If you choose to, that's fine. Perfect Posture will keep those hulking muscles toned when you're not flexing them. This program will only take what God has given you and make it properly proportioned and evenly toned.

## Crouching again

The line between getting Perfect Posture and keeping it is blurry. Therefore, crouching is included again. It will help you understand its importance both to **get** Perfect Posture, by finding where your center is, and to **keep** Perfect Posture through continued practice. By practicing, you make yourself more familiar with the inner feeling of when your body is centrally positioned. With practice, it becomes automatic in everyday life so Perfect Posture can be maintained. Refer to Chapter Four for detailed instructions and reasons for this important movement. No visualization provided with this one.

Do a crouch.

## Centering the Head

Judging by the number of complaints you hear about sore necks, how to center the head on the neck and shoulders is an appropriate topic for this book. A balanced head is essential for uncomplicated and complete recovery from an unbalanced activity, equipment load or injury. Two methods will be included.

### Balloon visualization

First, be sure your neck is as relaxed as your back. Touch the top, or central axis, of your head where illustrated in chapter two. Imagine your head attached to a large balloon right at that point. As the wind would blow the balloon out of vertical center, your hanging head would go with it out of vertical center. When the wind stopped blowing, the balloon and your head would drift back, into the vertically centered position. Visualize this in and out

**Image 7.01**
**Visualizing your head hanging from a balloon.**

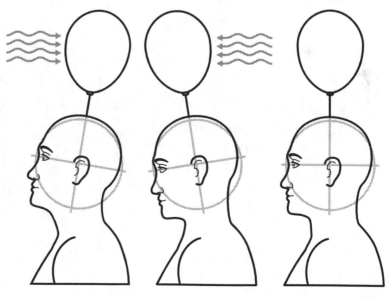

movement, finding the centered position frequently, until it becomes a habit. It can be done anywhere. Sitting or standing anywhere, you can be conditioning your body for balance and health.

This is a good comparison for the entire system and the idea of fluidity or perpetual motion. Activities of daily living will always be swirling around, causing you to move out of center. Activities rise and fall like the wind. Let your head drift back to the centered position, as if being gently pulled by the balloon, each time an activity has pushed you out of center.

### Horizon visualization

Another method for finding the center of gravity for your head is to stand, or sit, and gaze at a distant horizon. Any old horizon will do. Lift or shake the head, as in a yes or no gesture. Let the head bob. You will notice that the eyes move automatically against the direction of the head. Your vision is kept focused on the horizon. Slowly reduce the head movements. When your head feels like it's on an even plane with your eyes, and they are not looking up or down out of the sockets, your head is centered. Concentrate on the feeling. Make it a habit. When combined with the commandments and other visualizations, neck strain will be gone. Your head will sit squarely, midline on your shoulders without any strain front or back. [Image 7.02]

Don't get fixated with this or any centering imagery. You must and always will be moving in and out of center. You may be sitting down talking to someone standing up. You may be

**Image 7.02**
**Using your eyes to help center your head.**

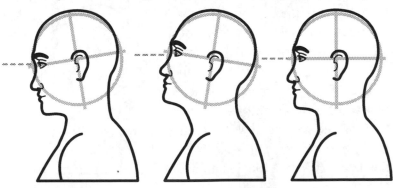

standing talking to someone sitting down. When they leave, or you leave, practice centering your head in the privacy of your own mind and body. **Then forget about it.** Go back to business as usual. In time, centering will be automatic.

## Centering the Shoulders

### Balloon visualization

Here's another balloon visualization, this one with your shoulders. Imagine two large balloons attached to the middle of the top of your shoulders. You're attached but the balloons don't pull up on your shoulders. They stay relaxed, sitting on your torso that sits on your unlocked legs. The wind blows the balloons forward, backward, side-to-side, whatever. Move your shoulders as if they were being pulled by the balloons in the wind. Now imagine that the wind has ceased and the shoulders gently return to their natural centered position. [Image 7.03] Repeat frequently so you get a feel for where your shoulders should be when at rest.

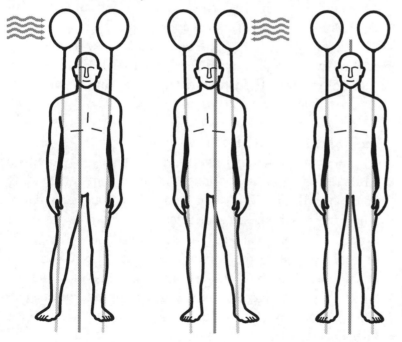

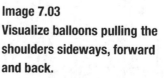

Image 7.03
Visualize balloons pulling the shoulders sideways, forward and back.

## Centering the Body

### Visualize riding in a boat

It's been said sailors love to dance. It's said they have a natural balance and rhythm. Come to think of it, have you ever seen an overweight sailor? It doesn't fit the stereotype. Could it be they spend a lot of time centering and burning calories when out in their boats?

Visualize yourself on a boat. A boat that's not too big, not too small. Don't make yourself uncomfortable. The movement of the boat on the water causes an unstable surface. It becomes necessary to stand in the biologically correct or Perfect Posture manner. [Image 7.04] If you tried to stand in the culturally appropriate manner, you would constantly be thrown off balance because your body is locked into a rigid, unnatural distribution of forces. Knees unlocked, constantly maintaining equilibrium is what you must do. If the water was very rough, it would be necessary to further lower the crouch in proportion to the roughness of the water. For everyday activities on solid ground, or calm water, slightly bent knees are appropriate.

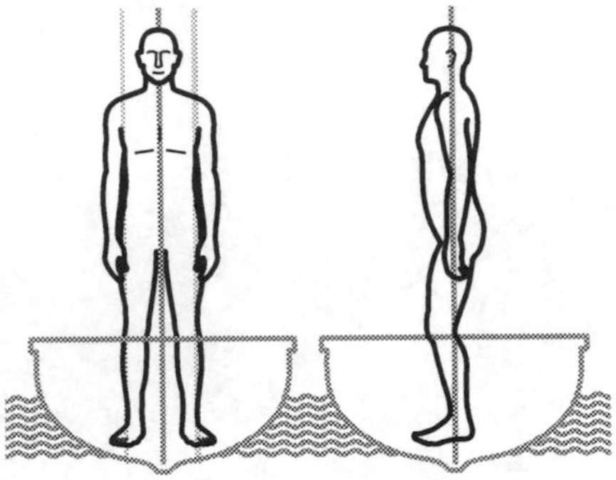

If the legs get tired or quivery, don't lock your knees to rest. You will cause unbalanced stresses which ultimately create deformities. Fidget, shift leg to leg and sit down, if you can. Slouch if you can when sitting.

**Image 7.04**
**Riding in a boat.**

**Image 7.05**
**Riding in a bus.**

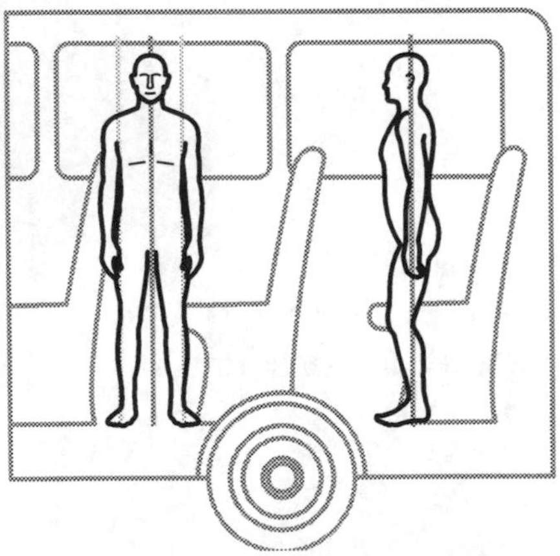

### Visualize riding in a bus

Some may remember the game of trying to stand up while riding on the school bus. Visualize yourself standing on the bus. [Image 7.05] You're trying to maintain balance while the bus brakes, accelerates, turns corners. In order to maintain your balance, you have to unlock your knees to better adjust to the forces exerted by the movements of the bus. If the bus was traveling very fast or cornering hard, you would have to hunker down more to have more control. For slow driving, everyday activities, keeping the knees barely unlocked will do.

### Visualize standing or walking on a large ball

At first it's hard. You need to stand in a crouch. As you practice, it becomes easier. You can straighten up some.

In time, poise and balance become second nature. It may take a while but, like any habit or hobby, with practice it becomes smooth, easy and automatic. You could stand on that ball all day and not get too tired. The concept should be getting clear. Learn to carry yourself in a manner as if the surface were unstable. [Image 7.06]

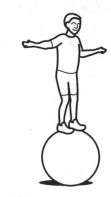

**Image 7.06**
**Standing on a ball.**

### Visualize standing or walking on ice.

When you first walk onto the ice, your hands may be out for added balance. As you got used to it, you could relax and let your hands drop to your sides. [Image 7.07] As your balance, poise and confidence increased, your hands would drop. Maybe even put them in your pockets.

In time, your legs would get used to the position and you could stand for longer and longer periods. Get too tired? Sit down. Butt gets cold? Get up and walk according to the commandments. Don't give in and lock your knees. You'd be deforming your body with each passing moment.

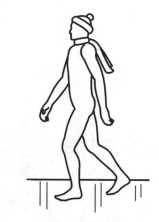

**Image 7.07**
**Walking on ice.**

### Visualize dancing.

How often do you see a professional dancer that's obese? Never? Just like with the sailor — it doesn't fit the stereotype. Pretend you're dancing. Stand like a dancer stands when waiting for the music to start. When you walk, develop the smooth transfer of weight that a dancer has when moving. Dancers don't plop from foot to foot while doing their steps. Do you hear a lot of thumping feet at a dance hall? Most dancers don't even know they're practicing Perfect Posture when dancing — but they are. They're never locking their knees when they dance and they can dance all night. Sure they get tired. They sit down to rest. If they're smart, they slouch. [Image 7.08]

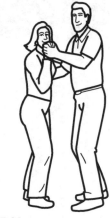

**Image 7.08**
**Dancing.**

## Spending Money and Setting Aside Time
## to Practice Perfect Posture

If you don't feel good unless you spend money and inconvenience yourself, exercise machines do the same thing Perfect Posturing does. I don't really like plugging someone else's product but, I really should point out the good aspects of these machines and gadgets. All of the following machines, and others too numerous to mention, almost force you to adopt Perfect Posturing body mechanics when using them. This is because their surface is unstable. Some have handles that help keep you from standing rigidly upright. Some even have handles that pull your shoulder forward with the opposite ankle during walk-like movements. You can use these machines almost indefinitely without becoming exhausted. You can burn a lot of calories using them – just like practicing the Perfect Posture gait.

My whole problem with an exercise machine is this: Why spend all that money, find someplace to conveniently store it, put all the time aside to use the thing, go through the bother of getting the machine out, setting it up, taking the time to use it, taking it down, then taking time to conveniently put it away? Too bad the machines aren't as convenient as your mind and body.

Wouldn't it be easier (and cheaper) just to visualize using the machine in your everyday life? Visualize the machine and use your mind and body. Make it a habit. You would get the same benefits and skip all the hassle. You could be applying the same body mechanics. You could mimic the same movements (unnoticeable when accelerated and unconscious) and be achieving the same results. Everywhere you went, everyday, all day. In reality you would simply be practicing Perfect Posture gait and skipping all those real problems with those real machines. Think of the money and time you'd save.

> A rose by any name is still a rose. Perfect Posture positioning by any method is still Perfect Posture positioning.

## Some Popular Exercise Machines

Notice how the dynamics of using these machines compels the user to maintain proper points of centering. You just about have to keep your knees unlocked and adopt Perfect Posture or you would lose your balance and fall off. If you have one of these machines, internalize the body mechanics while using them. Use those same body mechanics always. Get all the benefits of an unstable surface without the machine and hassles. Get those benefits all day, every day, practicing Perfect Posture. Really!

### The Gazelle.

This one makes you practice the Perfect Posture gait when you use it. The handle pulls the shoulder forward with the opposite ankle (see walking commandment #4.) It's almost impossible to lock the knees. Internalize the feeling. Walk that way when you get off the machine. Walk that way always. It would have the same benefit as being on the machine. Always, and everywhere you went, it would be like exercising on the machine. Sell it and just continue to walk that way. Visualize using it for practicing Perfect Posturing. You'd get used to it. Your body would become, or stay, properly proportioned and evenly toned all by itself. [Image 7.09]

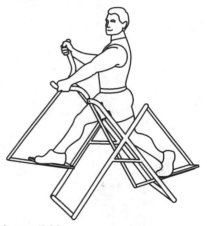

**Image 7.09**
**The Gazelle machine.**

### The stair stepper.

The dynamics of the machine, with its unstable surface and handles, just about force you to maintain proper structural hygiene. Use it to become familiar with keeping your knees unlocked and the body's feel when centered during locomotion. [Image 7.10] Or, sell it and practice some of the free visualizations previously listed. Or, sell it, walk up some stairs and internalize the feeling. Use a modified, accelerated form for your everyday, everywhere, all the time gait. Same difference.

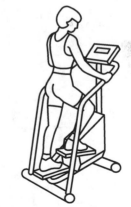

**Image 7.10**
**A stairstepper machine.**

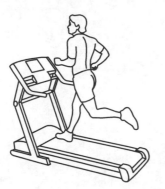

**Image 7.11**
A Treadmill on which the figure is carrying himself too upright.

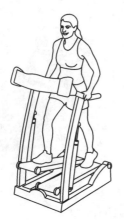

**Image 7.12**
A Treadclimber

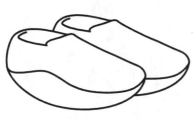

**Image 7.13**
Special Shoes

### The treadmill.

You almost have to keep your knees unlocked and assume a balanced position because the surface you're walking on is unstable and uphill. The treadmill could be used as a centering exercise to help familiarize your body's awareness of its center. [Image 7.11] Then, visualize using it whenever you walk. It would be the same movements. It would be the same benefits.

### Tread climber

Feels like you're walking on sand, it's said. [Image 7.12] Why spend all that money to feel like you're walking on sand? Just walk like you're walking on sand, for Pete's sake! Go to the beach and practice. Buy a pile of sand or steal some from the beach. Make a sandbox and walk around in it for practice. Get used to the feeling and walk that way. It won't look odd in everyday movement when your pace is accelerated. It's got to be cheaper than buying a machine. Get used to the feeling and walk that way. Practice your Perfect Posture gait when you go out to chase the cats out of it.

### Special shoes

Consider walking in shoes with hard rounded soles. They make them. The surface would be unsteady. You would be forced to keep your knees unlocked and maintain a centered posture to keep from falling over. [Image 0.13] Buy them, (they're advertised to get rid of cellulite.) Or *visualize* wearing them and save a few bucks. Walk that way. Get rid of your cellulite while you're at it.

Of course, your gait and posture will be exaggerated when you're practicing any of these visualizations. That's the way you want it. In fact, over-exaggerate when practicing. Of course you'll lose the exaggeration when you accelerate your movements during everyday activities. When you start, it will be noticeable to others that know you. But sooner or later, you'll get used to it. They'll get used to it. It will feel and look natural. You'll hear remarks about how good you look.

This is the end of the visualizing drills. Think up some others, possibly unique to your life and situation. How about these? Except for the walking during an earthquake, any of them could be visualized and done all day. You could even *really* do some. Pay for them and set aside time to do them if that's what you need. While really doing them, why not try to remember the feeling and stand and walk that way always? You'd get tired, but you get tired standing and walking in your straight, rigid, locked-up manner too. Practice frequently so it becomes automatic, unconscious in everyday, accelerated movement.

- **Standing on a rocking chair**
- **Walking inside a big ball**
- **Roller-skating or ice skating**
- **Standing or walking during an earthquake**
- **Cross-country skiing**
  **(Is this the gazelle in real life?)**
- **Standing or walking in a giant exercise wheel**
  **like a hamster uses**
- **Walking up or down an escalator**
- **Standing or walking on a bumpy plane ride**
- **Standing or walking on a trampoline**

# Chapter Five
# How to Keep Perfect Posture
## Part Two:
## Awareness/Time Chart

As you go about the day, it would be good to make a list of your posturing patterns in everyday activities. The questions and your answers in this chapter will give you an idea of where you stand in regard to habits that are giving you a not-so-perfect body. They will give you an idea of the time and concentration your counter efforts must involve. You can then respond with a pattern of progressions, crouches and balancing visualizations to counteract the unbalanced habits you've identified. In time, these progressions, crouches and visualizations will become habits and replace your previous unbalanced behaviors. It's like riding a bike, juggling or playing a musical instrument. Common sense tells you that if you don't give up and you keep practicing, the more familiar and comfortable these new patterns will get. Soon you'll be walking, talking, looking around, maybe even juggling or playing a musical instrument while unconsciously practicing Perfect Posture.

Use this time awareness section to help you think of what you will be doing and how you will best stay as close to center as possible during your day. Make copies and use them daily, to remind yourself to take a second to practice centering, or to plan the duration of a progression. Over time, the seconds will turn to minutes, minutes to hours, hours to days, days to months, months to years, and years to decades. That will add up to a lot of "credit" time on your postural account sheet. In time, you will be practicing Perfect Posture without even thinking of it. In time, you will *have* Perfect Posture without even thinking of it.

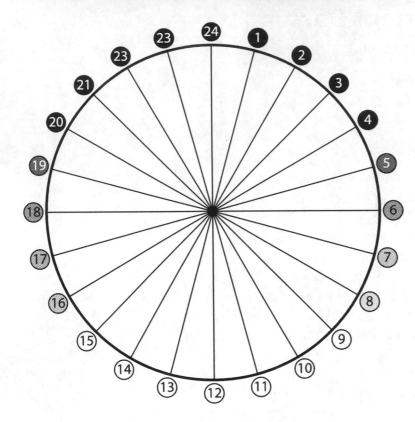

**Incorrect posture?**

When is my posture incorrect? *(Color in times when posture is not centered.)*

How is my posture being altered?

_____

Can I stand correctly in the situation I'm in?

_____

What amount of progression and/or visualizations are needed for correction?

_____

_____

_____

_____

_____

_____

If you have a job where you will be standing stationary in any manner, such as assembly line worker, start out unlocking your knees for short periods. Start out slow. Otherwise you will make yourself tired, burn-out and give up on the whole idea. This book will end up discarded, stored with the other exercise equipment in the garage or put out at the next yard sale. Remember, this is a way of life. Concentrate a little, get a little benefit. Concentrate a lot, get a lot of benefit. Do anything to keep from locking your knees to rest. Fidget leg to leg with knees unlocked. Get another job where you at least move a little.

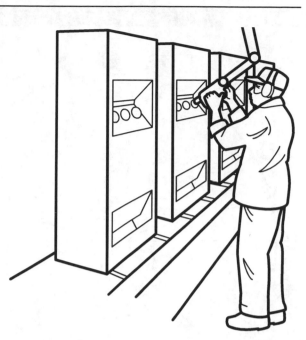

**(Check or fill in spaces that apply.)**

**How long will I be on my feet today? Hours_____ Minutes_____**

**What will I be doing while on my feet? Walking _____ Standing _____
Bending over _____ Lifting or carrying heavy objects _____**

**Will I lock my knees while standing or walking? Yes_____ No_____ If yes, how long____**

**What will I be wearing? High heels _____ Flat shoes_____
Somewhere in the middle? _____**

**How long will I be sitting today? Hours _____ Minutes_____**

**What position will I be in while sitting? Up straight _____Reclining _____
Somewhere in the middle _____ Will the position be? Steady _____ Intermittent _____**

**Will I be wearing anything that will make head support a challenge? Yes_____ No_____
How long? Hours_____ Minutes_____**

**Will I be subject to severe gravitational loads such as bouncing while operating heavy equipment or flying jet aircraft? Yes_____ No_____Hours_____ Minutes _____**

*(Fill in the above information so you can plan counteractive stretching progressions, crouches or visualizations to familiarize yourself to the centered, maximum recovery position. Add a question if needed.)*

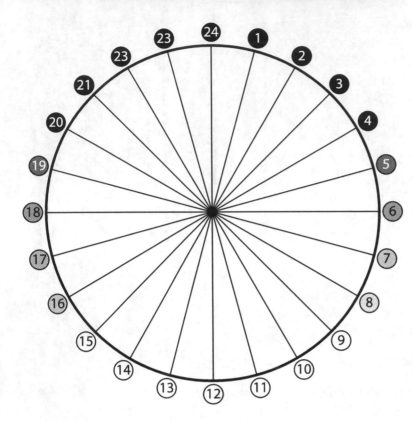

**Incorrect posture?**

When is my posture incorrect? *(Color in times when posture is not centered.)*

How is my posture being altered?

_____

Can I stand correctly in the situation I'm in?

_____

What amount of progression and/or visualizations are needed for correction?

Walking for a living is no better for your posture than just standing in a stationary position, if done incorrectly. Before beginning to walk, practice a crouch if you can and walk from that pre-descent position you learned with the shoulders above the knees. From earlobes to anklebones sense the centering points. It may sound tedious or exhausting but, your body was built for this. As time goes on, it will become second nature, balanced by nature. Toned and formed by nature. Don't snap the knees to the locked position with each forward stride. Keep the shoulders even with the opposite ankle. Practice in slow motion so it will carry over to accelerated, everyday movement.

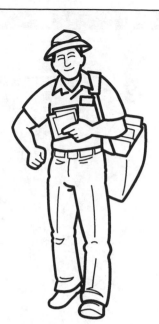

**(Check or fill in spaces that apply.)**

**How long will I be on my feet today? Hours_____ Minutes_____**

**What will I be doing while on my feet? Walking _____Standing _____ Bending over _____ Lifting or carrying heavy objects _____**

**Will I lock my knees while standing or walking? Yes_____ No_____ If yes, how long_____**

**What will I be wearing? High heels _____ Flat shoes_____ Somewhere in the middle? _____**

**How long will I be sitting today? Hours _____ Minutes_____**

**What position will I be in while sitting? Up straight _____Reclining _____ Somewhere in the middle _____ Will the position be? Steady _____ Intermittent _____**

**Will I be wearing anything that will make head support a challenge? Yes_____ No_____ How long? Hours_____ Minutes_____**

**Will I be subject to severe gravitational loads such as bouncing while operating heavy equipment or flying jet aircraft? Yes_____ No_____Hours_____ Minutes _____**

*(Fill in the above information so you can plan counteractive stretching progressions, crouches or visualizations to familiarize yourself to the centered, maximum recovery position. Add a question if needed.)*

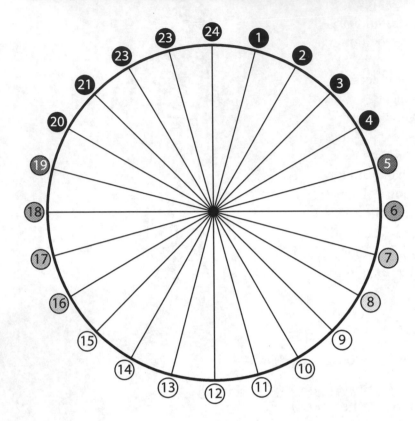

**Incorrect posture?**

When is my posture incorrect? *(Color in times when posture is not centered.)*

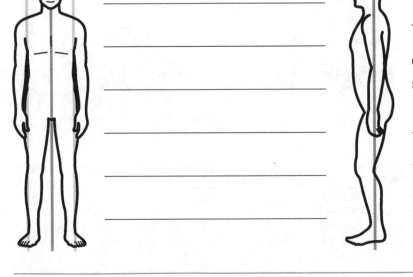

How is my posture being altered?

_____

Can I stand correctly in the situation I'm in?

_____

What amount of progression and/or visualizations are needed for correction?

Human bodies were created to hunt and gather, not repetitively lift heavy objects. Bending over, especially bending over and lifting, is very bad for the back and, therefore, posture. Bad for the entire body structure, for that matter. This is widely recognized today as evidenced by those people you see picking up litter on the side of the road with the fingers on a stick. If you are not one of those lucky people with fingers on a stick and you have to bend over and lift, the more aggressively you will have to act on the associated exercises, #1, #2, and #3 (carefully) for correcting the results of this occupation.

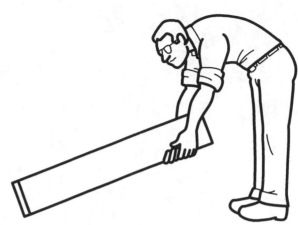

**(Check or fill in spaces that apply.)**

**How long will I be on my feet today? Hours_____ Minutes_____**

**What will I be doing while on my feet? Walking _____ Standing _____
Bending over _____ Lifting or carrying heavy objects _____**

**Will I lock my knees while standing or walking? Yes_____ No_____ If yes, how long_____**

**What will I be wearing? High heels _____ Flat shoes_____
Somewhere in the middle? _____**

**How long will I be sitting today? Hours _____ Minutes_____**

**What position will I be in while sitting? Up straight _____ Reclining _____
Somewhere in the middle _____ Will the position be? Steady _____ Intermittent _____**

**Will I be wearing anything that will make head support a challenge? Yes_____ No_____
How long? Hours_____ Minutes_____**

**Will I be subject to severe gravitational loads such as bouncing while operating heavy equipment or flying jet aircraft? Yes_____ No_____ Hours_____ Minutes _____**

*(Fill in the above information so you can plan counteractive stretching progressions, crouches or visualizations to familiarize yourself to the centered, maximum recovery position. Add a question if needed.)*

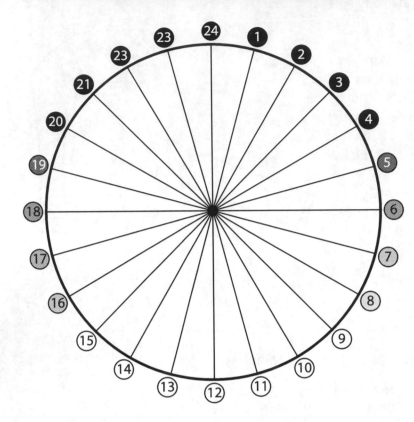

### Incorrect posture?

When is my posture incorrect? *(Color in times when posture is not centered.)*

How is my posture being altered?

_____

Can I stand correctly in the situation I'm in?

_____

What amount of progression and/or visualizations are needed for correction?

If you're a secretary and are required to sit at a desk all day in a straight-backed chair, it's very hard on your back. You're racking up postural debits. You're getting shorter. Your spinal disks are deforming. The pitch of your vertebrae is changing. See if you can get your boss to spring for a reclining chair and one of the keyboards you can place on your lap. Let him know about the positive effects: Less risk of carpal tunnel injury, less worker's compensation time paid, lower insurance rates for worker's comp. coverage. If he won't do it, get another job. You can get another job. You can't get another body.

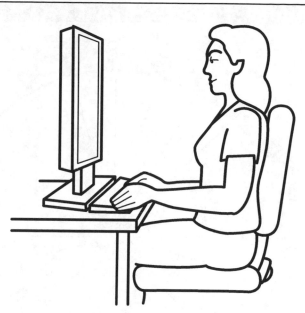

**(Check or fill in spaces that apply.)**

**How long will I be on my feet today? Hours_____ Minutes_____**

**What will I be doing while on my feet? Walking _____Standing _____ Bending over _____ Lifting or carrying heavy objects _____**

**Will I lock my knees while standing or walking? Yes_____ No_____ If yes, how long_____**

**What will I be wearing? High heels _____ Flat shoes_____ Somewhere in the middle? _____**

**How long will I be sitting today? Hours _____ Minutes_____**

**What position will I be in while sitting? Up straight _____Reclining _____ Somewhere in the middle _____ Will the position be? Steady _____ Intermittent _____**

**Will I be wearing anything that will make head support a challenge? Yes_____ No_____ How long? Hours_____ Minutes_____**

**Will I be subject to severe gravitational loads such as bouncing while operating heavy equipment or flying jet aircraft? Yes_____ No_____Hours_____ Minutes _____**

*(Fill in the above information so you can plan counteractive stretching progressions, crouches or visualizations to familiarize yourself to the centered, maximum recovery position. Add a question if needed.)*

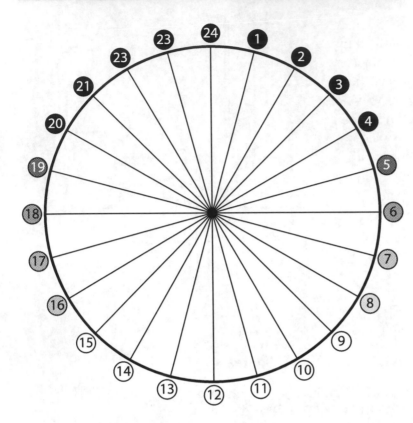

**Incorrect posture?**

When is my posture incorrect?
*(Color in times when posture is not centered.)*

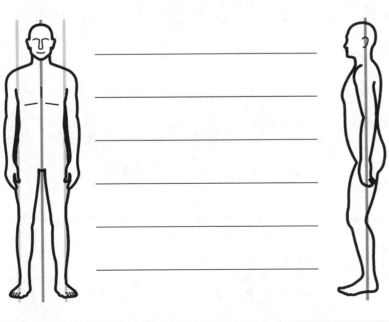

How is my posture being altered?

_____

Can I stand correctly in the situation I'm in?

_____

What amount of progression and/or visualizations are needed for correction?

Some jobs may be worth the hassle or are just plain essential. If you have a well-paying job, fun job or one that is essential no matter how uncomfortable or damaging it may be, you should be especially aware of its effects. You should be especially aware of Perfect Posture for ultimate recovery. This is because most likely it will require the most heightened level of alertness and peak physical condition to perform. Yours or someone else's life may depend on it. You should be especially aware so you're not functioning at suboptimal level. Especially aware so you don't have to retire early due to work related injury.

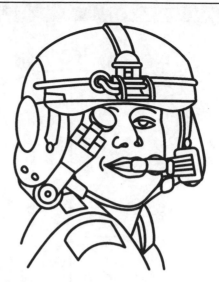

**(Check or fill in spaces that apply.)**

**How long will I be on my feet today? Hours_____ Minutes_____**

**What will I be doing while on my feet? Walking _____ Standing _____
Bending over _____ Lifting or carrying heavy objects _____**

**Will I lock my knees while standing or walking? Yes_____ No_____ If yes, how long_____**

**What will I be wearing? High heels _____ Flat shoes_____
Somewhere in the middle? _____**

**How long will I be sitting today? Hours _____ Minutes_____**

**What position will I be in while sitting? Up straight _____ Reclining _____
Somewhere in the middle _____ Will the position be? Steady _____ Intermittent _____**

**Will I be wearing anything that will make head support a challenge? Yes_____ No_____
How long? Hours_____ Minutes_____**

**Will I be subject to severe gravitational loads such as bouncing while operating heavy equipment or flying jet aircraft? Yes_____ No_____ Hours_____ Minutes _____**

*(Fill in the above information so you can plan counteractive stretching progressions, crouches or visualizations to familiarize yourself to the centered, maximum recovery position. Add a question if needed.)*

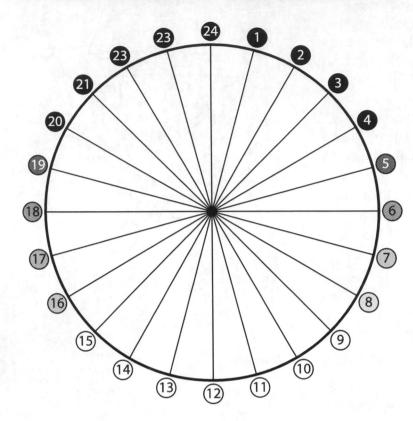

**Incorrect posture?**

When is my posture incorrect? *(Color in times when posture is not centered.)*

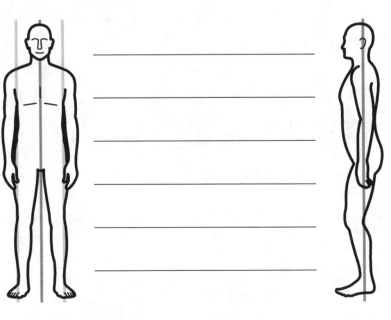

How is my posture being altered?

_____

Can I stand correctly in the situation I'm in?

_____

What amount of progression and/or visualizations are needed for correction?

So you've got the weekend off. Lucky you. Might go four-wheeling and pound your back for a few hours. It's the best. Take the speedboat out and bounce around on the lake, bay or ocean for a few hours. What a blast! Spend the day riding horses. Sounds like fun. Take a long drive. Get your mind off things. Work in the garden. It's so relaxing. Clear the back 40. It's got to be done. These activities may be rewarding, but, pure heck on your back and body. Just remember Perfect Posture principles and progressions when you're done. It takes time to ruin your back and posture. Don't be caught wondering how it happened.

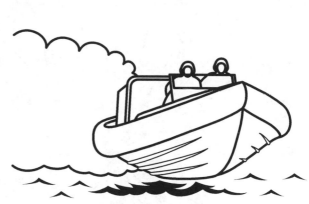

**(Check or fill in spaces that apply.)**

**How long will I be on my feet today? Hours_____ Minutes_____**

**What will I be doing while on my feet? Walking _____ Standing _____ Bending over _____ Lifting or carrying heavy objects _____**

**Will I lock my knees while standing or walking? Yes_____ No_____ If yes, how long_____**

**What will I be wearing? High heels _____ Flat shoes_____ Somewhere in the middle? _____**

**How long will I be sitting today? Hours _____ Minutes_____**

**What position will I be in while sitting? Up straight _____ Reclining _____ Somewhere in the middle _____ Will the position be? Steady _____ Intermittent _____**

**Will I be wearing anything that will make head support a challenge? Yes_____ No_____ How long? Hours_____ Minutes_____**

**Will I be subject to severe gravitational loads such as bouncing while operating heavy equipment or flying jet aircraft? Yes_____ No_____ Hours_____ Minutes _____**

*(Fill in the above information so you can plan counteractive stretching progressions, crouches or visualizations to familiarize yourself to the centered, maximum recovery position. Add a question if needed.)*

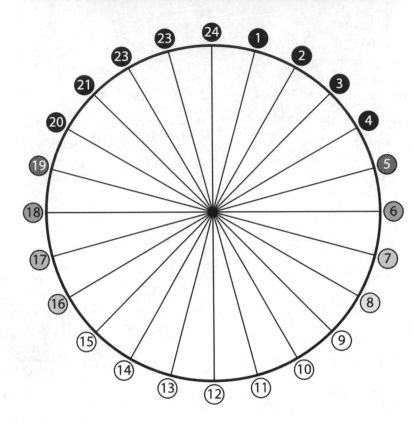

## Incorrect posture?

When is my posture incorrect?
*(Color in times when posture is not centered.)*

How is my posture being altered?

_____

Can I stand correctly in the situation I'm in?

_____

What amount of progression and/or visualizations are needed for correction?

Another day off? Lucky again. Take it easy today. Kind of sore from yesterday. Start off at church. Sit in the straight, hard seats. Then a ballgame or a movie. Concert or play, anyone? May have to stand in line for a while but it's worth it. If you stand with your knees locked, you're damaging your spine and posture. Spilling your guts, creeping yourself out. Unlock those knees. Align your points. Shift foot-to-foot, lean, dance the box step. After standing, you'll sit on hard bleachers or a straight chair for another few hours. If you can't slouch, you're buckling your spine. At the least, assume position #1, as tightly as comfortable, when you get home.

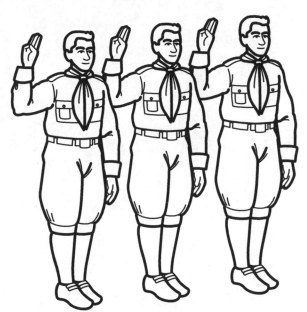

**(Check or fill in spaces that apply.)**

**How long will I be on my feet today? Hours_____ Minutes_____**

**What will I be doing while on my feet? Walking _____Standing _____
Bending over _____ Lifting or carrying heavy objects _____**

**Will I lock my knees while standing or walking? Yes_____ No_____ If yes, how long_____**

**What will I be wearing? High heels _____ Flat shoes_____
Somewhere in the middle? _____**

**How long will I be sitting today? Hours _____ Minutes_____**

**What position will I be in while sitting? Up straight _____Reclining _____
Somewhere in the middle _____ Will the position be? Steady _____ Intermittent _____**

**Will I be wearing anything that will make head support a challenge? Yes_____ No_____
How long? Hours_____ Minutes_____**

**Will I be subject to severe gravitational loads such as bouncing while operating heavy equipment or flying jet aircraft? Yes_____ No_____Hours_____ Minutes _____**

*(Fill in the above information so you can plan counteractive stretching progressions, crouches or visualizations to familiarize yourself to the centered, maximum recovery position. Add a question if needed.)*

## A Final Word

You now have the knowledge and tools to keep a Perfect Posture for your entire life. The world can always use more poise and quiet strength. Be one of them. Or be loud with Perfect Posture. You can be whatever you want. If you're older, you can look the same as when you were young and probably better. If you're young, don't lose any time standing incorrectly. The longer you have poor posturing, the harder it is to change your habits, the harder it is for your body to reshape itself. If you have children, teach them the proper body mechanics so it's a habit early on.

It may be hard in the sense of breaking a bad habit and starting a new one to replace it. Not hard in the sweaty, monotonous, exertion sense. But it will be worth it. You can be properly proportioned and evenly toned by nature, front to back, side to side and top to bottom with the simple effort of habit. It will be a habit done without thinking after it becomes a conditioned response.

— David Paul

Printed in the United States
by Baker & Taylor Publisher Services